Toilet as Business for the Hygiene of the Chinese Community in Colonial Hong Kong

Yuk-sik Chong

Toilet as Business for the Hygiene of the Chinese Community in Colonial Hong Kong

Springer

Yuk-sik Chong
The Chinese University of Hong Kong
Shatin, Hong Kong

ISBN 978-981-19-1395-2 ISBN 978-981-19-1396-9 (eBook)
https://doi.org/10.1007/978-981-19-1396-9

This Springer imprint is published by the registered company Springer Nature Singapore Pte Ltd.
The registered company address is: 152 Beach Road, #21-01/04 Gateway East, Singapore 189721, Singapore

Acknowledgements

From the early 2010s, when I first began thinking through my ideas to research public toilets in Hong Kong, I have accumulated many debts of gratitude to institutions and friends. My debt of gratitude is especially large to the Hong Kong Institute of Asia-Pacific Studies at the Chinese University of Hong Kong, which supported me in rewriting my Ph.D. thesis from which this book derives. Various libraries and archives kindly granted me access to their materials. The following were particularly considered: Hong Kong Public Records Office, the Museum of Medical Science of Hong Kong, Po Leung Kuk Archive, Tung Wah Hospital Archives of Hong Kong, the University of Hong Kong, and the Chinese University of Hong Kong.

I would like to especially thank the following people for encouraging and helping me in the course of my work on this research. Among them are Tai-lok Lui, Xiaoli Tian, Ho-yin Lee, and Shun-ching Chan at the University of Hong Kong, Gary Hamilton at the University of Washington, Wan-tai Zheng at the Chinese University of Hong Kong, and Koon-yiu Ma, Wing-mei Yu, Sun-pao Ting. In addition, my special thanks to Krzysztof Jankowski, who reads the manuscripts and enlightened and challenged me, helping me to sharpen my ideas in the complexity of urban governance in colonial Hong Kong. Last but not least, this book is dedicated to my family, with love and thanks.

Hong Kong
August 2021

Note on Romanization

It is impossible to standardize the romanization of Chinese words, as Hong Kong speaks Cantonese, but not Mandarin, the national language of China. For easy reading, the romanization of Chinese names and terms from Hong Kong is primarily based on Cantonese pronunciation, such as Ho Kai rather than He Qi. Place and institution names in Hong Kong are also in Cantonese romanization, for example, Wanchai and Tung Wah Hospital. However, a few famous names and terms are given in pinyin, such as Soong Hing Ning and Sun Yat Sen, as they are already known to many readers by those spellings. Names from China are either in the long-used English rendering or are in pinyin, in line with Chinese national practice. For example, Guangdong is used rather than Kwangtung (in Cantonese). Treaty names are listed according to contemporary standards, such as the Treaty of Nanking.

Contents

Abbreviations

AJPH	Address of the Excellency Sir John Pope Hennessy to the Legislative Council
AR	Administrative Report
BB	Blue Book
BPP	British Parliamentary Papers
CM	China Mail
CRN	Contract for the Removal of Night Soil from Public Privies
CSR	Colonial Surgeon Report
DWF	District Watch Force
FoC	Friends of China
GG	Government Gazette
HKDP	Hong Kong Daily Press
HKH	Hong Kong Hansard
HKRS	Hong Kong Records Service
HKT	Hong Kong Telegraph
HKWP	Hong Kong Weekly Press
MSB	Minutes of Sanitary Board
PLK	Po Leung Kuk
RB	Rate Book
RCHK	Restrictions Upon Chinese at Hong Kong
SCMP	South China Morning Post
SP	Sessional Papers
SSR	Sanitary Superintendent's Report
TKP	Ta Kung Pao
TWH	Tung Wah Hospital

List of Figures

List of Tables

Chapter 1
Introduction: A Mix of Profit Accumulation and Regulation of Urban Space in Toilets

> An old brick building of 2 floors, open to external air on 3 sides, 16 windows, but as they are kept closed the light and ventilation is bad, brick and tile foot-rests, zine buckets (some defective) cement floor good, channels to square cement-lined cesspool inside building.[1]

1.1 Overview

Between 1860 and 1930, most sanitation infrastructure in colonial Hong Kong was provided using large public toilet facilities supported by the government and wealthy Chinese. Public toilets are defined as toilets that could be accessed by the general public; regardless of charging a fee or being free of charge, they may be owned and operated by the government or private sector. Such toilets were in fact commercial operations supported by "toilet economies" of facility leases (typically twenty percent higher than residential),[2] patron entry fees (one or two Chinese copper cash),[3] and the selling of the collected feces-night soil-as fertilizer on the open market. In toilet economies, the emerging world economy's impact on local urban governance became clear, and the pail system was the common form of toilet in the colony prior to the Second World War (1941–45), where night soil was removed by hand, which was viable only as long as the night soil could be sold to the nearby silk industry in southern China.[4] In turn, such a regional silk industry relied on global demand, as European colonial powers and the United States needed larger quantities than they could produce themselves. From silk, the world economy gave value to the human waste being deposited in public toilets, which facilitated the government and Chinese business to establish and commercialize toilets to discipline lower-class Chinese in using urban space in order to prevent open defecation, albeit mediated by profits. As the colonial discourse of urban hygiene invoked a fear of environmental and moral threats, the disease originated from the waste of this class of Chinese people.[5] Both government- and privately owned toilets were commercial toilets operated on a quasi-commercial basis, and their placement and operation were characteristic primarily of night soil collection points. By 1899, the number of public toilet seats was split

Y. Chong, *Toilet as Business for the Hygiene of the Chinese Community in Colonial Hong Kong*, https://doi.org/10.1007/978-981-19-1396-9_1

75/25 percent (531/173 toilet seats) between private and government ownership in Victoria City, the primary urban area in Hong Kong at the time (stretching from contemporary Causeway Bay to Kennedy Town).[6]

The new governance rationality, based on capitalism, introduced an aspect of maximization of interests in the quest for continual profit accumulation to maximize the use of urban space, increasing the complexity of regulating space. That public toilets were business ventures operated by the government and business necessitates a political economy approach in which market influence came to directly interfere and reshape government-led efforts to "civilize" lower-class Chinese living in Hong Kong. This approach is used to show how the sanitation regime emerged out of a complexity of contestation and collaboration between the government and Chinese business elites (night soil contractors, privately owned toilet operators and toilet landowners), balancing the regulation and profit maximization of urban space. Through prominent Chinese politicians, business contestation took place through government public toilet site negotiation, questioning whether the government had a monopoly on public health and the moral role of government toilets in urban hygiene. While the weight of collaboration was founded upon racial and class politics, the requirement, rationale, rebuttals, and arguments in favor of the toilets were bound up with night soil and land interests and an imagery of the lower-class Chinese as a race-apart, whose dirty habits were the source of disease that threatened urban order, which was held by both the government and business. Through providing the majority of toilets, business elites became a strategic partner to the government in the exercise of control over their fellow countrymen.

In a market-oriented system, the approach of the government to toilets was, however, heavily economic, that its presence in the night soil business and land market was an impetus for entangling health services with economic interests and engaging business resources in regulating lower-class Chinese, thus reordering urban space to be civilized, moral, hygienic, ordered, and profitable through toilet provision. Unable and unwilling to fund a comprehensive sanitation system itself, the government was forced to enlist business elites to provide the toilets that would ultimately come to govern lower class Chinese everyday hygiene behavior. Such a collaboration and the overall commercial operation of sanitation infrastructure went against the colonial moral discourse of urban hygiene. This discourse was derived primarily from a moral order of urban space, which sees toilets purely as morally charged spaces for the government to discipline local society's defecation practices, inducing the right kind of sanitary habits.[7] Such a change would be towards a moral lifestyle of conformity and behavioural self-regulation so that the goal of an orderly city could be achieved through self-regulation of bodily behaviour rather than through coercive measures.[8]

A capitalist turn of sanitation does not imply that the government was moral, and business was just; in fact, both hoped to fulfill their own competing concerns in one place. This is also done with no intention to place capitalist concerns over moral concerns. Rather, it examines the complex political and economic interactions between government and business and the changing pattern of governmental spatial regulation in response to land and night soil profits. This is reflected in multiple internal divisions of class within Chinese, European, and the government over sanitation, which contradict the dichotomy of colonizer and colonized, of which assumed a binary and hierarchical spatial relationship in regulating urban space, that the toilets functioned as the everyday metaphor of colonial discipline over urban space. The contradictions provided clues to the new spatial relations that were being reconstructed between capitalism, space, and morality (self-regulated and governed one's own hygiene behaviour). That toilets were commodified and their role as night soil collection points being maximized brings insights into a new moral geography that blended moral and capitalist logics within sanitation infrastructure. This displays how each party's interest—urban space regulation and profit accumulation—came to be enacted in the toilets, so moral and capitalist logics were worked upon lower class of Chinese. Toilets were honed to be night soil collection points that generated maximum profits and helped to remove defecation from urban space and could better respond to some of the major dilemmas of urbanization and urban regulation within capitalism. In a capitalist system, there is a conflict emerging between space as a means of production, generating profit from urbanization that often leads to increased land value,[9] and the resulting urban growth (reflected in the population and rubbish) that quickly worsens urban conditions, such as poor sanitation.[10] While relieving the sanitation problem requires establishing urban order in cleanliness through the regulation of space, that process can threaten the profit accumulation process.

The engagement of government in the night soil business and land market and the capacity of business, especially Chinese landowners, in reordering urban space are highlighted in the analysis, both with reference to internal and external economic developments. It was evident that the commercialization of sanitation and the economic interest ethic of capitalism drove the government's and business's urban governance efforts of public toilets. Following Jon Pierre's definition of urban governance as the "processes through public and private resources are coordinated in the pursuit of collective interests",[11] this government-business collaboration in Hong Kong was a joint mobilization of resources. To sketch out the mode of urban governance in this capitalist colonial context, this analysis highlights the transformation from governing through a hierarchical order to one of collaboration, that the colonial government and Chinese business had informally exercised some forms of resource (land and regulatory capacities) exchanges to achieve the task, reordering space. What was the governance model through which the government and business governed the colony? How did the two parties mutually constitute and actualize each other's political and economic interests? What were their strategies for achieving the task of reordering space and generating profits, and how effective were they? In this analysis, the author will be concerned with the business interplay of contestation and cooperation with the government over sanitation and the changing role and capacity of business in governing the colony. Moreover, the nature of resource exchange and the formation of a moral-capitalist mode of governance are based on a particular set of interests and values.

Modeling the moral capitalist mode of governing space is valuable to unravelling the complexity of regulation and profit maximization of urban space and contributes to the analysis of urban governance in colonies in two significant ways. First, the emerging public toilets were night soil collection points within a world system of deep functional and geographical divisions of labor and purpose—colonies and semicolonies (e.g., China, which was partially occupied by a variety of colonial powers), as peripheral areas, supplied resources such as night soil to serve core colonial powers' demand for silk. This brought toilet provision into interaction with the world economy, shaping colonial Hong Kong local governance. Second, land is a critical resource that was overlaid with the contradictions and tensions between spatial regulation and profit accumulation embedded in the colonial capitalist system and contextualized within Hong Kong's political economy. By capturing the competing discourses of urban hygiene through the multiple internal class divisions over sanitation between pairs, such as the governors and the colonial military force, sanitarians and government administrators (and Chinese politicians), and Chinese business elites and lower-class Chinese, these discourses urged the inclusion of capitalist interests within sanitation infrastructure. Such changes were bound up with the local, regional, and global economic developments, bringing profit directly into the racial dimensions of toilet provision. Toilets as urban space mean that the means of production were governed not only by the logic of morality but also by profit making.

Considering the relationship between capitalism and the form of government spatial regulation, public toilets towards the regulation of space (containing human excrement and restricted defecation in confined and private areas) provided an illuminating analytical window through which to examine the changing character of infrastructure (from purely moral space to the blending of capitalist logic into the infrastructure) in urban hygiene, which was mediated by profit. By providing the convergence of moral and capitalist logics to the theoretical discussion on new moral geographies that blended with capitalist interests, this analysis shows how the government interacted with Chinese business elites in reordering space, with an emphasis on the interplay of contestation and consensus among competing discourses of urban hygiene. This change in the elite Chinese public role involved an intersection of morality, space, and capitalism: "toilet economies", which sustained toilet services, that bought out how Chinese interacted with the government and was involved in governing the colony. This analysis provides insights into how colonial public health responses were impacted by the emerging capitalist economy of the nineteenth century, and three major issues will be discussed in this book as follows.

1.2 World-System and Colonial Urban Governance

Silk, night soil and public toilets seem unrelated, but they were all linked in nineteenth century Hong Kong within the global economy. Interlinked by trade, such an economy is a world system divided into core, semiperipheral, and peripheral areas based upon the mode of production—the type of technology and organization of labor used.[12] In the modern world system of the nineteenth century, the core countries were distinguished for being colonial powers with economic and military hegemonies, superior technology and capital-intensive production. The semiperipheral and peripheral countries were mainly colonies (including semicolonies) with inferior technology and economies founded on labor-intensive production and resource extraction. These economies were forcibly delegated to supplying raw resources and products to core economies to meet global consumer demand. This rooted the world economy in capitalist logic, which divided the world by a division of labor determined by the functional relation to capital accumulation. The world was to be understood as a set of economically interdependent societies. Often, we see analyses of world capitalist development premised upon nations and cities; however, very little study has been carried out on how world-system linkages shaped the mode of urban governance in colonies. This study is concerned with analyzing the increasing importance of silk exports to the world market in China's economy, pushing Pearl River Delta farmers (located in the southernmost province Guangdong, which is near Hong Kong) to increase mulberry tree cultivation rapidly from 1860 to 1930, leading to the public toilet market in Hong Kong. It must be noted that this is not a detailed study of China's silk industry development within the world system, and there are many existing studies on this topic.[13]

1.2.1 *The Linkage of Silk, Night Soil, and Public Toilets*

It is necessary then to extend our view beyond local conditions when looking at urban governance in colonial Hong Kong. It emerged from the periphery, and its public toilets served as peripheral-economic units: supplying a raw resource—night soil—for China's own semiperipheral economy that supplied silk to meet the demand of core industrial and colonial powers. China's silk had long been famous for its high quality, and its products became part of the export trade of the Ming dynasty (1368–1644).[14] After the First Opium War (1839–42), the silk industry was widely linked with the core powers' silk markets, meaning that massive exports of silk to Europe and the United States ensued, especially from the late 1860s onwards.[15] Particularly, when the European colonial powers and the United States became industrial powers, their purchasing power increased, including their demand for luxury goods such as silk and tea.

The link of China's silk industry to core markets dramatically increased the regional demand for night soil used to fertilize mulberry trees for silkworms. Adding to the demand for Hong Kong night soil in particular, it was believed that urbanites' excrement was better quality, owing to their diet consisting of more protein than the typical rural peasants' diet, which was mostly vegetarian.[16] This meant urbanized Hong Kong's night soil was preferred in China. The premium paid for Hong Kong night soil made it attractive to sell, up to HK$0.70 a picul (one picul equals about sixty kilograms) in China in 1899, while the collection price in the colony was HK$0.28 a picul by 1898, meaning the profit was significant.[17] Thus, from the late 1860s, early in Hong Kong's colonial development, a cross-border night soil business developed between the colony and nearby Shunde, the main silk-producing area in the Pearl River Delta of Southern China.[18] Here, the issues are as follows: In what ways did the defeat of China by the colonial powers speed up the incorporation of Hong Kong's local governance into the world economy? Why did incorporation begin in the 1860s?

Economics was central to toilet provision across all countries (including colonies) prior to the twentieth century, as governments that attempted to provide toilets were always thwarted by underfunding.[19] At the time, it was common to turn toilets into commercial sites (through selling night soil or toilet paper or charging an entrance fee) to fund the service. As a valuable economic commodity, selling night soil generally generated profits from either local or regional economies.[20] Inspired by Douglas's notion of dirt,[21] we see that whether night soil is considered to be "a matter out of place" depends on where it is situated. The famous Chinese phrase "night soil is gold" best illustrates its value in agriculture. For all its value, the night soil sitting in toilets might also have been gold, and that value enabled toilet services to be financially sustainable.[22] There have been many studies examining economic factors in toilet provision, but relatively few connect to the wider impacts of capitalist development. This lack of connection in the analysis prevents us from understanding what impact the incorporation of colonies into the world system had on toilet provision. For Hong Kong, the geographical profit source of public toilets spanned local areas, China, and the world. This applied a mixture of micro- and macroeconomic opportunities and pressures on public toilet provision. As a vast agrarian country, the trade of night soil is particularly attractive in China.[23] The increasing demand and value for night soil for mulberry trees drove Hong Kong night soil contractors to collect it, pushing the development of a citywide network of toilets to collect night soil from across the colony.

Toilet operators drew revenue from two sources: selling night soil and charging an entrance fee. This dual income meant operators were willing to pay high toilet rents to landowners, who were mainly Chinese. Landowners leased their properties as privately owned toilets from the late 1860s up to the early twentieth century.[24] At first glance, at least five of these landowners were compradors: Choy Chan's son Choy Kwai Ng (Messieurs Hotz S'Jacob & Co.)[25]; Kwok Acheong (Peninsular and Oriental Steam Navigator Company) and his son Kwok Yung Kam (Ying Kee Company)[26] Ng Sang (Douglas Lapraik & Co.) was also a partner in Wong Li Cheng Hong, which exported Chinese silk and tea to Britain[27] and Pow Ping Kwan (Olyphant & Co.).[28] However, toilet economies were not limited to government and Chinese business, and transnational European companies such as Jardine Matheson & Co. (British conglomerate) and Siemssen & Co. (German conglomerate), which possess huge land resources, were also interested in leasing their properties as toilets. However, only three privately owned public toilets were operated between them. The former owned one at 13 Tai Wong Street, Wanchai, from 1882 to 1895, while the latter owned two at 6 Tak Hing Alley East, Saiyingpun, from 1870 to 1895, and 5 Po Yan Street, Taipingshan in the early 1870s.[29] Such a citywide network of toilets was basically developed by the government and Chinese business in a market relation characterized by toilet economies.

In the nineteenth century, the public toilets were primarily intended to be used by lower-class male Chinese. There were two factors: first, the public toilets for common use were against Chinese culture, because females could not expose their body in public[30]; and second, the majority of the Chinese who fled to Hong Kong to earn a living were male. The ratio of male to female was approximately 75% to 25% before 1900.[31] While higher-class male Chinese did not need to patronize these toilets, as they were allowed to use more hygienic pail toilets in restaurants, and had adequate night soil buckets at home. Similarly, Europeans of different classes could use toilets (both pail and water closet) in European company premises and hotels. By 1880, there were 182 water closets, mainly situated in European company premises, homes and hotels.[32]

1.2.2 Urban Governance Between Government and Chinese Business

In seeing attractive profits, the government also began tendering the night soil deposited in its own public toilets in 1869.[33] Government toilets became not only economically self-sufficient, but they actually generated considerable revenue for the government, on average approximately one percent of total yearly government revenue between 1869 and 1930.[34] As public toilet profits depended on the night soil's manurial value (a key factor of continuing toilet services), night soil served as a strong weapon of resistance for Chinese business to the authority's disinfection requirements,[35] affecting government-business relations and their strategies in reordering space. Indeed, toilets were a valuable urban property that existed in a symbiotic relationship with the countryside; farmers purchasing night soil with manurial value generated funds for sustaining toilet services in the cities, creating a sanitary equilibrium as urban waste was exported and farms fertilized.[36] What was the role of government in the night soil business, and how did this change the political nature of night soil? What form did the cooperation between night soil contractors, toilet operators, toilet landowners and the government take in the capitalist turn of sanitation in relation to the global silk market and local land market development? These questions provide insights into the operation of colonial economies and the characteristics of colonial rule in terms of sanitation. They should be examined in the study of colonial urban governance of public toilets; however, they have rarely been addressed in colonialism studies or public health.

The financial sustainability of the public toilets provided by both the government and business corresponded with various prevailing economic and political circumstances in Hong Kong and the world, including the supply and demand of night soil and silk, disease outbreaks (1894 plague outbreak in Hong Kong) and the enactment of major public health ordinances (*the 1887 Public Health Ordinance*). Commercial demand for night soil entangled capitalism, morality and urban space together, significantly impacting colonizer-colonized and government-Chinese business collaborations in reordering space. In this scenario, urban governance was exposed to, and so highly affected by, the global economic restructuring occurring at the time. The impact of the favorable silk market is an important focus of the analysis. The silk trade made urban governance between the government and business possible but also put the availability of toilets at the mercy of regional night soil and global silk markets. The government-business collaboration over toilets operated through the interplay of three markets: land, silk, and night soil. Therefore, it is not a surprise that toilet landowners and toilet operators withdrew from the toilet market when Chinese silk-producing regions were devastated by local floods and global silk demand was greatly reduced by the Great Depression in the first two decades of the twentieth century.[37] This caused a drastic reduction in the number of privately owned toilets, from eighteen to thirteen between 1899 and 1905, further decreasing to eight and two by 1920 and 1930, respectively.[38]

Therefore, the world-system perspective offers a synopsis of one place's urban governance becoming increasingly intertwined with the evolving global economic contingences. The emergence of Chinese business's public role in governing urban hygiene occurred along with the capitalist turn of sanitation. In terms of the international division of labor, this book will examine in what way did a favorable world silk market affect China's silk industry and night soil market and the sustainability of Hong Kong public toilet services? How did emerging global capitalism make toilets such a profitable business venture, leading to the colonial government and Chinese business jointly regulating lower-class Chinese bodies and their use of urban space? Furthermore, how did cooperation with the government that came out of this economic reality facilitate Chinese business leaders to gain a greater role in urban governance? As business acted with the government to comanage lower-class Chinese, we are required to ask what global economic conditions interacted with regional silk and night soil markets and local land markets to influence this government-business method of urban governance. Second, we need to ask, how did the political and economic conditions of the nineteenth century generate novel alliances across racial and class boundaries, which ultimately came to redefine the nature of sanitation infrastructure? These questions are key to understanding how the world system impacted local urban governance and colonial spatial order.

1.3 The Formation of a New Moral Geography

Under the influence of a capitalist world economy and land market, there were complex government-Chinese business interactions over urban regulation, which had important impacts on blending capitalist concerns with moral ones within public toilets. Toilets worked both as a moral space and as a means of production that blended not only moral and capitalist logics but also racial and class politics. Spatial ordering was complicated by a mixture of capitalist, colonial, and ethnic forces under capitalism, which were further complicated by the contingent urban development and regulation of a rapidly growing colony. This challenged the perceived spatial order of colonial authority and moral discourse of urban hygiene, forming a new moral geography. A focus of this analysis is the changing form of spatial regulation that began to emerge. This was a shift from simple segregation of disorderly space and designation of morally charged spaces to creating spaces that implicated moral order and economic concern. Such spaces regulated the lower-class Chinese public defecation and the use of urban space, which were considered to cause disease by the government and Chinese business.[39]

1.3.1 Dirt and Disorder

Urbanization became a new challenge in the modern world as it brought dire sanitation risks and disease that repeatedly devastated cities, significantly raising death rates, even giving birth to the idea of the spatial relation between disease and environment. The relation was specifically highlighted in a report about the sanitary condition of the Hong Kong working class population in 1842 by Edwin Chadwick, the first British Sanitary Commissioner, who argued that miasma originated from unhygienic bodies and spaces, spreading disease.[40] It was believed, in the nineteenth century, that diseases occurred from exposure to miasmas. Bashford further elaborated the relationship that "disease was understood to be a response to decomposing, putrefying matter in the surrounding environment—human waste, accumulation of dirt, stagnant water, foul air. The latter was understood as the main medium of transmission".[41] Based on the miasmatical theory, it was suggested fecal emanation might cause disease and infection, it was not only confined to direct contact but also through the inhalation of foul air from decomposed human waste, by visiting the public toilets or living in the vicinity of the toilet, for example.[42]

Rather than just a fear of the actual diseases that the waste could cause, there came to be the fear of disorder. Douglas explains how dirt and disorder are connected: "If we shun dirt, it is not because of craven fear, still less dread or holy terror. Nor do our ideas about disease account for the range of our behaviour in cleaning or avoiding dirt. Dirt offends against order".[43] Dirt in public gained the symbolic meaning of being situated beyond its proper boundary, being "matter out of place" and so was morally besmirched, incongruent with urban order and civilization. By the mid-nineteenth century, the discussion of dirt (such as human waste) in Europe was becoming increasingly associated with civilization.[44] Levels of civilization came to not only represent the advancement of technology, but manners in the self-consciousness of bodily control which involved an increase in shame; not blowing one's nose or defecating in public were considered matters of civilized order.[45] The dirt in public association with disorder and disorders' own association with loss of bodily control were deemed dirt to be judged as immoral. As proper placement is associated with morality, dirt creates a spatial boundary between profane and sacred, and the exclusion of profane from urban space provides a mechanism to protect the sacred from contamination conceptually (morality) and physically (body).

The institution of the boundary between dirt and clean was then essential and had a profound effect on colonial urbanism in which there was a hierarchical distinction between sanitary and insanitary in lifestyle and sanitary behaviour along racial lines,[46] leading to the establishment of spatial boundaries between indigenous and European spaces (posited as civilized, hygienic, and orderly) being drawn in colonial cities, including Hong Kong.[47] Most notably, the colonial notion of dirt ran along racial lines and was closely interwoven with a fear of lower-class Chinese lifestyle and hygiene behaviour causing disease and contaminating European morality. The most significant occasion was the outbreak of "Hong Kong fever" in the summer of 1843, and 440 deaths out of 1,526 troops were recorded in that year.[48] However, the most terrible statistic is that there were 7,893 cases treated in the hospital, as each man, on average, contracted the disease more than five times. The high death toll and repeated hospitalization alarmed the government, which located disease within the inherent improper lifestyle of Chinese, so that a link between the health of Europeans and the garrison with that of the lower-class Chinese and their areas was established.[49]

Therefore, there was an urgency to manage the use of urban space emerged partly due to the spread of real disease and partly because urban hygiene was increasingly associated with urban order. The fear of disease and moral contamination provided a means for the government to reorganize space, which drove to regulate Chinese people's bodies and their habitation of urban space, entailing a segregation that meant they were marginalized to the lower-western part of Victoria City in the 1840s.[50] "Sanitation syndrome" is the term coined by Swanson to depict this understanding of colonial spatial relations; sanitation syndrome justified urban segregation based on hygienic behaviour rather than race,[51] which became a colonial policy to regulate Hong Kong urban space and the lower-class Chinese.

1.3.2 The Morality of Public Toilets

Regulatory responses to urban space-maintained general sanitation include the designation of a space as morally charged, mediating the relationship between bodies and space. Public toilets were designed to regulate bodily waste to organize urban space, as technology grew more advanced during and after the Industrial Revolution in the West, the notion of moral and racial supremacy of whites burgeoned.[52] This supremacy was increasingly associated with the idea of civilization and brought an increasing importance of public toilets to urban order, in that defecation had to be performed in toilets that were enclosed and ensured dirt was kept in its proper place.[53] Defecation and deposited waste in toilets, which prevented transmitting disease and endangered urban order, were perceived to be civilized lifestyles and constructed as an issue of morality.[54] By providing a confined and private area for defecation, toilets created the essential controlled conditions of an ordered structure with a well-designed internal spatial organization for the government to nurture moral well-being. Moral governance was built into the physical structure of the toilets so that an ordered toilet space (achieved through the clean and white spaces that facilitated illumination made these structures more visible and ordered, which were associated with cleanliness and morality, while also facilitating a clear line of sight for observation and management, allowing the government to create social norms among toilet users' and attendants' hygiene behaviours that helped maintain sanitary conditions.[55]

Founded on a new, highly ordered kind of space, the standard of norms could be formulated, and any deviation could be easily identified. The norms set a tone of disciplined behaviours shared by society that was underpinned by the judgement of right or wrong, which had constraining effects on people to conform to it. This involves the concept of morality, resting on the idea of making people accountable for their actions, which was important to creating a hygienic urban environment. This was a system of self-regulation against the old form of knowledge, which was based on coercion or legal regulations, in which the government replaced coercion with moral regulation that worked on the "conduct of conduct" through the regulation of space.[56] This new form of governance focused on the self-discipline of the people under the guidance of the government. Through such guidance, the capacity to regulate oneself as a disciplined body could be developed in a manner whereby people were not coerced into stopping undesirable behaviours and could effectively enforce cleanliness and urban order. This means that morality could be developed from within rather than being coerced by external restraints. Toilets became a locus of moral governance regulating bodily habits, within which a sense of self-regulation could be instilled among people, bringing cleanliness and moral order to urban space. In discussing how toilets served as a morally charged space which reordered urban space in Victorian Britain, Brunton, Hamlin and Wright describe the toilet interiors were well lit and ventilated (free of miasma which is regarded as diseases), which had a practical function to help toilet users and attendants see what they were doing and others were doing as well, which could regulate behaviour and introduce moral habits to people, for the protection of urban space.[57]

Within the framework of colonial governmentality, it is important to recognize that there was a hierarchical moral order in colonies, but rather than simply exercising authority over urban space, colonial governments designated spaces (structure or built environment) as colonial milieus, subject to the machinery of authority to which the government could arrange things in a logical order and manage dangerous bodies (e.g., disease producers), thus protecting urban order.[58] Then, the designated space would serve as a moral geography to instil moral qualities in people to move towards a moral lifestyle and use urban space properly. Caused by the view of moral difference embedded in racial politics, public defecation was believed to be a part of locals' chosen culture; they were seen as unable to control their orifices and thus required enclosed toilets to contain bodily waste.[59] However, Anderson argues that colonial public toilet provision in the Philippines was not simply driven by various colonial government obsessions with 'matter out of place'—of bodily waste deposited in public—but also a concern for disciplining unhygienic local bodies by close surveillance.[60]

Similarly, more than pragmatic, public toilets were also constructed as a rationalizing instrument of moral governance on the everyday life of the colonized in Hong Kong. We will see why public defecation was seen as moral corruption of the lower-class Chinese and became an increasing concern of the colonial authority after the 1850s, which was not only treated as being dangerous to sanitation but also disorderly.[61] After a series of disease outbreaks led to extraordinary garrison mortality in the mid-1860s, the British parliament became alarmed, which led the Hong Kong government to urgently seek a way to introduce public health measures such as public toilets to contain bodily waste and improve urban hygiene in 1867.[62] Following this, the government curbed public defecation and legislated proper night soil collection and disposal methods in the same year.[63] The public toilets were a particular focus of the former Royal Engineer Osbert Chadwick's investigation in 1881; he was the son of the first British Health Commissioner Edwin Chadwick.[64] His investigation report best illustrates that toilets were perceived by the government as a colonial milieu introducing habits of cleanliness to lower-class Chinese.

1.3.3 Land Capitalism and Public Toilets

However, as noted earlier, government public toilets accounted for only 25 percent (173 seats) of the total public toilet seats in Victoria City by 1899, meaning private toilets were the dominant contributor to general sanitation. The good profits attracted Chinese businessmen, who had the market sense to operate a citywide network of privately owned toilets sustained by an industry of night soil contractors, toilet operators and toilet landowners with income generated from selling night soil, charging toilet entrance fees, and leasing the properties. The marketization of toilets intensified when the land market was connected with the night soil business and the silk industry. Well aware that night soil was a profitable enterprise—contractors offered a good price to collect night soil from operators who were willing to pay high rents—and landowners were extensively involved in the public toilet market in return for higher rental returns than residential uses from leasing properties as privately owned toilets. These toilets came to be the dominant toilet system, creating a functional dependency by the government on them for sanitation services in lower-class Chinese areas, saving public funds and land while avoiding conflicts stemming from intervening in Chinese daily life as promised by the colonial government.[65] This raises the question: how did the government and Chinese business get caught up in this complex, and sometimes antagonistic, arrangement?

This peculiarity is exacerbated as the arrangement arose between the contradictions of moral regulation and profit accumulation of urban space, as well as racial and class politics in a capitalist system. In Hong Kong, the focus on land capitalism was inextricably linked to the rise of the land market in the restructuring of the economic system due to self-financing since the colony opened in the 1840s.[66] This had a unique feature in the high land price policy; government revenue was then focused on auctioning land parcels that were rationed to attain the highest price possible, creating a market of very scarce, and hence valuable, land. To ensure high revenue, land was sold at auction, and the increasing population caused an appreciation in the value of land. There was a 60% rise between mid-1854 and mid-1855, houses were in such high demand that 100 new houses were constructed, and another 200 were under construction.[67] This especially attracted heavy investment from Chinese people in the land market, which in turn boosted government revenue.[68] Land revenue accounted for 10.7–31.3% of total yearly government revenue over the period of 1878–1910.[69] Land revenue was a vital income source, along with the opium monopoly, before the early twentieth century.[70] The institutionalization of the land market promoted property investment while tightly integrating revenues into the government financial system. Hence, the analysis will explore how elites and administrative officials reshaped approaches to public health under the conditions of world economy and capitalism.

Noting the capitalist fervour over urban space, Chattopadhyay argues that the emergence of the land market in colonial India stirred capitalist dynamics and challenged the prevailing racial spatial order, redefining the colonial government's designated use pattern of space.[71] Indeed, land profits played a core element driving government-business collaboration in Hong Kong urban governance of public health. The impacts were expressed in two ways. First, the introduction of a land market created the conditions for maximizing land interest among both business (Chinese and European) and administrative officials, which engaged a contest to colonial urban hygiene moral discourse by them that public health should be concerned with economic interests. The multiple internal class divisions among Chinese, European and the government became contradictory to the dichotomy between colonizer and colonized over sanitation, creating opportunities for government-Chinese business collaboration in toilets, which fulfilled each other's interests.

That Chinese business captured the entanglement of public health and economic interests to challenge the discourse by using Chinese culture and the importance of land revenue in the colony, reformulated what they perceived as misunderstanding of urban hygiene and argued that Chinese landowners and privately owned toilets could also take up public role in reordering urban space.[72] Tensions between the regulated and profitable control of urban space also occurred within the government (e.g., between the Sanitary Board and the Public Works Department) and the Europeans (e.g., between the ruling class and landed class) over the provision. For example, on the basis that a land parcel would generate an estimated HK$60,000 at auction, a proposal made by the Sanitary Board to build a toilet close to Belilios Public School was opposed by the Public Works Department and thus cancelled.[73] It is evident that the complex interaction between the key players was one of conflict and cooperation, interplayed by racial and class politics in a capitalist system. This analysis asks, how did different key players respond to the challenges of urbanization and capitalism in the realm of public health? Answering this question examines how the capitalist class divisions that formed facilitated government-business collaboration in the market turn of sanitation, which led to a major modification in sanitation infrastructure's spatial configuration. The Chinese business elites and officials contested prevailing moral hygiene discourses and turned public toilets into a means of production by producing hybrid forms of sanitary infrastructure.

1.3.4 *Public Toilet: A Place of Hybridity*

These spatial contradictions (the entanglement of capitalism in the public health-restructure para) that were driven by the influence of capitalism are clearly seen in early Hong Kong public health provision, specifically the entanglement of government and business in land interests. Such contradictions led to multiple internal class divisions over sanitation, providing market-driven service provision in which the availability of toilets was left to market forces. Moving beyond the fact that government and business were in competition over urban space, or the hierarchical spatial order between government-business and colonizer-colonized, the book focuses on colonial collaboration and the new capitalist spatial order. How did these factors create a new set of power relations within the government itself and between it and Chinese in urban governance? First, we shall see how contesting the moral discourse of urban hygiene lay at the heart of land-centred capitalism and was endemic to Hong Kong as a new governance, the maximization of profits increasing the complexity of regulating space. This was reflected in the logic of the new moral geography, which was complicated by a mixture of capitalist, colonial, and ethnic forces through public toilet provisions. What tensions between colonial government and Chinese business in controlling urban space and the profit of urban space marked this geography? How were these tensions further complicated by the largely unplanned urban development of a booming colony and the aim of regulating lower-class Chinese bodily waste? Such questions illustrate the colonial and urban complexities that interplayed the political and economic tensions between the government and business over the regulation and profit accumulation of urban space, contributing to our understanding of the moral capitalist mode of urban governance of public toilets.

Second, the presence of a capitalist form of governance rationality created a set of new and different conditions that meant local elites were obliged to act as active social agents in colonial policies.[74] This was, of course, the result of self-interest of both the government and Chinese business elites, who worked upon themselves toward a mode of self-governance of daily life, that however contributed to the urban governance between government and business and the public interests of the colony. In Hong Kong, the emergence of capitalist development created new conditions for capitalist expansion that were important to the rise of Chinese business elites, as their wealth and land resources grew, creating a condition of self-interest in toilet provision. They were obliged to involve themselves in the toilet market and govern urban hygiene to maintain their interests, as will be seen in the Chinese District Watchmen in supervising night soil removal from public toilets in the 1880s.[75] First, they benefitted from the "toilet economies". Offering public toilets for their lower-class Chinese tenants also reduced the pressure to offer toilets in tenements. The business heavily invested in land and built extensive tenements without toilets to maximize rentable space. Furthermore, embedded in racial and class politics, the colonial urban hygiene discourse invoked a fear of environmental and moral threats, which eventuated a belief among the Chinese elite class that the disease originated from lower-class Chinese bodily waste. With the imagery of a deficient lower-class

Chinese, there was rising concern about poor sanitation among the general Chinese community, manifested in the hierarchy of class and class interests (land profit).[76]

As hygiene became more associated with class, Kidambi and Rogaski are correct to note that both race- and class-shaped colonial urbanism, adding that local elites always shared their interests with the colonial governments in intervening in the daily life of their fellow countrymen.[77] It was in this convergence of racial and class interests that the moral and economic functions of toilets were achieved in Hong Kong, as they came to serve as a colonial milieu for managing bodily waste. This facilitated government-Chinese business interaction in marketizing the morally charged toilets and regulating lower-class Chinese, albeit mediated by "toilet economies" and land interests. This was critical, as it was important to both parties to exclude waste from urban space, thus maintaining clean neighbourhoods and property values that were needed for the colony to grow and increase the land revenue. Furthermore, the neighbourhoods in the Chinese quarter exhibited a fairly large degree of intermingling of classes, and the houses of the wealthy Chinese might be in the vicinity of these tenements.

Even though Hong Kong public toilets were operated in a quasi-commercial manner, they played a role in presenting the morality of toilets in public health. The commercial aspect was combined with control over lower-class Chinese bodily waste, facilitated moral governance of the government on these Chinese and displayed colonial authority in urban space. It can be said that these toilets, which blended moral and capitalist logics, were negotiated spaces between regulation and profit accumulation of urban space, as well as the colonial government and Chinese business. This is somewhat similar to how Bhabha describes colonial urban space as "a place of hybridity" lying between "inside" and "outside" and "inclusion" and "exclusion", constituted by contradictions between the government and the local society manifesting as cultural interactions.[78] Places of hybridity undermine the colonial ideal logic that was binary and hierarchical, while muddying assumed spatial relations. Such effects are characterized not only by political contestation but also by the creation of opportunities for colonial collaboration. It is within the context of this hybrid space, which involves negotiated meanings between profit and regulation, that the morality of public toilets could be approached through a combined strategy of well-designed physical structure and everyday surveillance with the support of laws and negotiating with business interests.

These toilets were clearly designed to a substantial extent in reference to a paradigm of urban order that privileged bright, hygienic and orderly environments.[79] For example, more ventilators were opened to increase the natural light and circulation of air and to minimize nuisance and enhance visibility, facilitating surveillance. These improvements were reinforced by a sanitary inspectorate system based on laws, together with relentless surveillance of everyday toilet behaviour, toilet cleansing and night soil removing practices, exerting pressure on proper behaviour and practices,[80] so that self-regulation among Chinese to maintain toilet cleanliness and urban hygiene could be developed. Equipped with law, Foucault argues that even though it cannot help but be armed, it can formulate norms giving government the powers to govern the people.[81] To ensure that hygiene was in good order, policing of urban space and toilets called for a standard set of public behaviours of night soil removal by coolies and of toilet cleanliness maintenance by attendants consisting of periodic disinfection, limewashing and scrubbing according to the 1867 *Ordinance for the Maintenance of Order and Cleanliness* and the Instructions to Head Watchmen and Watchmen, for example.[82] The task of policing was important; it symbolized the presence of agents of government that it was constantly undertaking surveillance.

Therefore, the regulation of urban space was thus not simply configured by the colonial authority on political grounds, but it was rather driven by economic interests from both the government and Chinese business. Under such conditions, business was able to sustain toilet services with economic strategies and reshape public health policies to their advantage by entangling economic concerns with the policies. That the public toilets worked both as a means of production and as a moralizing technology meant that they were representative of a new moral geography that blended moral and capitalist logics. These morally charged spaces fulfilled material and discursive purposes; practically, they could maintain sanitation and foster urbanization to further generate profit, mediating the dangers of human waste while maintaining a clean neighbourhood would facilitate the next round of urban development and profit accumulation. Discursively, these toilets helped reshape spatial relations and rebuild social order. The author will explore how capitalism became a new governing rationality through the examination of a set of socioeconomic conditions when Hong Kong was established as a treaty port in the 1840s. This examines the questions, why and how do the two logics coexist within toilets? How important was the coexistence to the economic sustainability of public toilets? How did government and business maintain their relationship in the daily operation of public toilets?

1.4 Land Resources: Interplay of Constraint and Facilitation

Toilet provision involved different players, and Chinese landowners were a distinct elite group highly involved in the toilet market.[83] The marketization of public toilets intensified when the land market became connected with the night soil business. This not only highlights a mode of business engagement shaped by land resources but also a complex interaction of urban contestation and collaboration with the government in urban hygiene. We shall see the land holdings of some prominent Chinese, who leased their property as toilets. Furthermore, they used these resources to oppose health proposals, which instrumentally helped them sustain their privately owned toilets. The heavy involvement of Chinese landowners was particularly critical in the colonial Hong Kong capitalist system. They were not only land-rich and economically powerful, being the top twenty taxpayers since the mid-1870s, but were also a group of emerging political (e.g., Legislative Councilors, the Justice of Peace, JP) and social elites (e.g., Directors of the Tung Wah Hospital, TWH and Po Leung

Kuk, PLK).[84] When land was increasingly concentrated in the hands of people with similar ethnic or social backgrounds, such resources were politicized, consolidating Chinese landowners' structural position in urban space regulation. This meant that these landowners were in a privileged position, determining who was eligible for hygiene facilities and their location. However, their significant role as a force in urban hygiene has been understated in the prevailing scholarship.

1.4.1 Urban Contestation

Many studies have identified land as the critical resource in providing sanitation infrastructure, but authors emphasize Chinese landowners' pursuit of capitalist interests, hampering proposals to improve public health.[85] There is some truth that capitalists, including landowners, are often the first group in society to work for their own class interests. 'Class-for-itself' is the term used by Marx to describe a class's self-awareness of their position in the relations of production and the purposeful agitation for change in their favor.[86] For Thompson, class "does not exist", rather class only occurs in cultural and social formations where consciousness arises from conflictual situations. He argues "class is a relationship, and not a thing", but rather, "happens when some men, as a result of common experiences (inherited or shared), feel and articulate the identity of their interests as between themselves, and as against other men whose interests are different from (and usually opposed to) theirs".[87] While the channels of personal connection are more closely tied to some political systems and economic structure of the society, which are more malleable to interest articulation among the people, so that people who have common social backgrounds (e.g., class, culture, and race) are more easily organized and so are more effective in interest articulation.[88]

In Hong Kong, the concerns of the colonial government were mainly centred on commercial development, which made it adopt a minimal intervention approach to Chinese daily life. This created a segregated social-political sphere between the government and general Chinese, which facilitated Chinese business elites to cultivate social influence among the Chinese community by offering the most required social services, helping them to mobilize resources (social capital) for their own interest in the name of protecting Chinese culture.[89] Indeed, this allowed business with land resources to articulate common interest among themselves and mobilize resources for their own class goals. The capitalist land system prompted landed-class elites to collectively use their land to compel the government to revise any public health proposals that threatened their land-sourced rewards. For example, in 1878, they opposed the proposal to require more illumination and air flow to their lower class Chinese tenants in tenement housing. This was done on the grounds that the government lacked an understanding of the unique Chinese living style (e.g., windows are kept closed for security reasons).[90] In another case dated 1887, public health was perceived as a symbol of British cultural imperialism incompatible with Chinese culture (e.g., women would not share toilets with tenants from a different family), so that the Chinese Sanitary Board member Ho Kai opposed the compulsory provision of domestic toilets in tenement buildings.[91]

It is very easy to see this as a zero-sum game that the government was compelled to make concessions to business by compromising public health under the pressure of socioeconomic forces.[92] It is also easy to assume fear of racial tensions between colonizer and colonized, being a particular concern in colonial contexts, urged the government to keep a distance from the latter's daily lives to avoid conflict, creating a policy gap for public services that Chinese elites filled.[93] There is some truth to these assumptions, but the mere adoption of minimal intervention, or political compromise, insufficiently explains why landed-class elites massively entered the toilet market. What has been ignored is that the agency and capacity (e.g., land resources and social capital) of these resourceful elites facilitated and sustained toilet provision more effectively than the government could. Studies that focus on private land power constraining public health proposals miss what role capitalist urban space could have in facilitating public toilet provision. The reordering of space was achieved with the help of Chinese landowners, who provided privately owned toilets for profits.

Instead of employing the conventional ways that put emphasis on the constraining aspect of land powers to limit public health implementations, the analysis examines their urban contestation with the government from an interplay of both constraining and facilitating aspects of land powers and how these landowners used their huge resources to provide toilet services, which made the government dependent on them for such service. That is, the control of land was the source of political power for Chinese elites in restructuring government-business relations over toilet provision. The enormous political significance of the concentration of land resources in Chinese landowners, including their impact on urban governance, is one of the main concerns of this analysis.

1.4.2 Public Function of Chinese Landowners

Seeing the public functions of business in a market-oriented system, Lindblom argues that the relationship between government and business in such a system is structured such that business needs incentives to perform the functions.[94] This is counter to following the traditional way that dependent on the interlocking relationship between the ruling class and capitalist class based on common social origins, the government moves towards a position of granting privileges (tax reduction, a say in government policies) to this specific class to induce public functions. Lindblom notes that the government clearly understands business function is indispensable, as the welfare of society rests in their hands. The government is obliged to share governance with business by granting them privileges to induce them to perform functions for the public interest. Considering the public functions of landowners in a market-oriented colonial society, their privileged role in urban governance and relationship with the government are greatly under researched. In Hong Kong, Chinese landowners performed the function of maintaining general sanitation by leasing properties as public toilets and sustaining toilet services through their huge land resources, which granted them a privileged position as partners with the colonial government in exercising control over lower-class Chinese bodily habits.

The heavy involvement of landowners in the toilet market is a result of Hong Kong's colonial economy, characterized by the centrality of land markets in government and business revenue and expenses. This coincidentally opened opportunities for Chinese to accumulate substantial wealth and land, creating a condition of self-interest to maintain neighbourhood cleanliness, increasing property value. As noted earlier, the Chinese elites built extensive tenements without toilets to increase rentable space, which also incentivized them to offer public toilets for their lower-class Chinese tenants to maintain general sanitation. Second, landowners seized a more general opportunity created by land scarcity, and they were well placed to provide the most needed resource—land—to privately owned toilet operators. This suited the government, as it saved it from building on crown land to supply sanitation infrastructure, so it could be auctioned, preventing the loss of potential revenue for the government. Third, drawing on their huge land holdings, elite Chinese could advantageously locate privately owned toilets among their other properties, thus controlling environmental complaints about miasma from other landowners. This formation of the "spheres of influence" allowed toilet services to operate in intensively populated locations for decades.[95] What were the patterns and development modes of the spheres? It is important to realize that the spheres were not operated independently; they involved a complicated social network between toilet landowners and other elites. The multilayered web of relationships through first personal ties and then business, social, and political links will be explored. How did the complex web of relationships allow landowners to contain complaints and provide toilets effectively, creating the government's functional dependence on them for sanitation services? Toilet site negotiations from landowners posed a major obstacle to the government's own efforts to provide toilets.

A model based on the facilitating aspect of land power is different from the constraining model in that it emphasizes Chinese landowners' agency to develop and sustain toilet services. Nevertheless, the term "facilitation" here is not a neutral term; it can be understood as a strategy by landowners for securing "toilet economies" and improving property values by minimizing bodily waste in the streets. It can be seen as the productive effect of land power. According to Foucault, power also has a productive aspect that operates through the production of new knowledge and discourses. It is well argued by Foucault that "if power was never anything but repressive, if it never did anything but say no, do you truly believe that we should manage to obey it?".[96] However, as mentioned, previous studies about land power mainly focus on the role of collusion, paying little attention to the productive aspect of the collaboration. Hence, this analysis not only examines urban contestation imposed on government toilets by landowners but also extends the focus to their involvement in a market-driven toilet program that, in one sense, "coincidentally" helped maintain sanitation. Through such a more dynamic approach, this enables us to better understand what the task of reordering space, done by government and Chinese landowners collectively rather than against each other, achieved.

It is interesting to know what types of landowners became involved in the toilet market. In what ways did they work with Chinese politicians in the changing discourse of urban hygiene? It is also important to keep in mind that the colonial government and Chinese elites were uneasy partners; they were collaborators in some aspects, rivals in others.[97] Therefore, how did landowners use land in a complicated manner to contest government toilets while sustaining private toilets at the same time? In answering this question, it is important to bear in mind that in supporting toilet services, landowners also made the provision of toilet services more capitalist (e.g., maximizing the night soil collection capacity by increasing toilet seat numbers) and political (e.g., as a negotiated space between government and Chinese business over the use of urban space). These landowners, in supplying and sustaining the necessary sanitation infrastructure, undertook a public role that transcended the spheres between government and business, colonized and colonized. What concerns this analysis is that Chinese as a whole altered their role from that of passive recipients to public service providers. The analysis will explore how such a change resulted in spear-heading colonial government-Chinese business urban governance and the spatial regulation of lower-class Chinese bodily waste, giving birth to a truly modern spatial logic of hygiene that did not accord with colonial urbanism.

1.5 The Development of Colonial Urban Hygiene

The capitalist-moral governance of sanitation emerged in nineteenth century Hong Kong under the influence of the world system, combining local and regional economic factors. Much has been written on the moralizing effects of sanitation improvements made possible by the hybrid toilet system, consisting of Asian night soil selling and Western sanitary management.[98] Little attention, however, has been paid to the emergence of the new moral geography and the consequent capitalist-moral mode of urban governance. Chinese business contested and cooperated with the colonial government in providing toilets and maintaining general sanitation while the government retreated from its role as a direct provider. This suggests that their relationship was not a zero-sum game but rather that it was more complex and interdependent. The participation of profit-motivated business in sanitation led to toilets becoming blended spaces of regulation and profit accumulation. By viewing moral space production within a political economy framework, we not only see contestation between government and Chinese business but also contestation within the government and amongst Europeans. This captures how the convergence of different parties' respective interests for regulation and profit accumulation were blended in the toilets and in the interaction between private interest and public good. This shows that capitalism, morality, and urban space were intertwined in complex ways, challenging the notion that toilets were merely profitable or moral sites.

In adopting the political economy perspective to public toilet provision, this analysis has three main new developments. First, it disentangles the complex colonial government-Chinese business interactions that worked to overcome the challenges of an urban colony in a world economy with respect to local, regional, and global markets. This not only accounts for how colonial urban governance was shaped not only by economic contingencies at the local level but also at the world level within the world system. Despite the many studies on the economic dimension of toilet provision or colonial collaboration in public services shown earlier, there has not been much enthusiasm to make the connection to the specific governance aspects of public health in a colonial society or to the wider perspective of the world system.

Second, political economy broadens the understanding of toilets as an overlapping space of regulation and profit accumulation that operated to meet both the competing logics of morality and capitalism. This accounts for how a mixture of moral and capitalist concerns was a spatial expression of government-local business collaboration that was integrated within racial and class politics. Together, such a mixture could more effectively maintain general sanitation in the capitalist colonial context. Most importantly, in toilet provision, it points to the convergence of profit and urban order, highlighting the competing discourses of urban hygiene. This leads to new insights into moral geography forms, that of the capitalist turn of sanitation infrastructure that nonetheless contributed to maintaining order.

Third, there is undeniable evidence that Chinese elites, especially landowners that were situated in a confluence of societal forces and huge land holdings, often worked as strategic partners of governments in terms of social control and urban development. The emergence of new economic developments in Hong Kong's local and regional vicinity and the world produced a new set of rules for Hong Kong governance. This generated conditions conducive to Chinese landowners taking up an ostensible public role in reordering urban space to secure their economic and class interests. This ostensible role converged with government and business engagement in "toilet economies" and the need to address public defecation by lower-class Chinese through public toilet provision.

Fully analyzing the development of urban hygiene in colonial Hong Kong requires going beyond political (the fear of disease that threatened urban order) and local factors (growing population and health crisis). The intimate connections among the global silk trade, China's silk industry and the land market within the world system, and their impacts on public toilet provision and local governance need to be unraveled. To this end, Chap. 2, "Political-Economic Conditions for Chinese Business Elites Taking a Role in Governance", begins the discussion by outlining the political-economic conditions for collaboration between the colonial government and Chinese business elites. Restructuring in the economy and tax systems offered opportunities for Chinese people to accumulate wealth and resources required to be involved in urban governance. This chapter examines the dynamic nature of government-business collaboration over public services, which is important to illustrating the public function of the business sector and the shared governance between them.

Chapter 3, "Governing Urban Space: Racial and Class Politics", discusses the fear of disease and how morality was projected onto toilet provision to regulate lower-class Chinese bodily waste and their use of urban space. Under the influence of capitalism, the multiple internal class divisions within Chinese, European and the government over sanitation were present in the governance of urban hygiene and spatial order, complicating the provision of sanitation infrastructure. It may help readers locate the tensions between urban regulation and profit accumulation in capitalism. The competing discourses of urban hygiene were constructed by different groups of social actors, which set the stage for the capitalist turn of sanitation and colonial collaboration over toilets, mediated by the market.

Following these two chapters, Chap. 4, "Toilet Economies: Night Soil Profit, Toilet Entrance Fees and Rent", proceeds to identify the new economic conditions of the nineteenth century world system that led to the inclusion of capitalist logic in toilet provision. This shows that the transformation of toilets into night soil collection points perfectly matched the colonial powers' rising silk demand, triggering both the colonial government and Chinese business elites to directly involve themselves in the night soil and toilet markets. Through that transformation, the chapter explores the extent to which toilet provision was linked to broader local, regional and global economic developments, showing how the world economy impacted local governance. Finally, this chapter examines the impacts of the government changing its role from being a direct service provider of toilets to that of a "market-friendly" government through facilitating night soil and privately owned public toilet businesses by providing pro-market measures.

In Chap. 5, "A Blending of Moral and Capitalist Logics in Public Toilets", the entanglement of capitalism, morality and urban space is examined. The capitalist turn of sanitation blended two logics, which formed a new moral geography that facilitated government-Chinese business collaboration over exercising control over lower-class Chinese bodily waste. This will be studied against the backdrop that some Chinese were able to attain an elite status based upon their landownership. Chinese landowners have employed a series of strategies to keep their busy public toilets open in dense residential areas for decades. At the same time, these toilets could not be kept open without government input (e.g., an inspectorate system to supervise night soil removal and maintain a minimum of toilet cleanliness, on the basis of legal framework). Its involvement was critical to the coexistence of moral and capitalist logics in the toilets; thus, the supportive role of government in granting privileges (e.g., tax incentives, no requirement for night soil disinfection) for business will be examined. As the government also had its own agenda, the privileges were thus subject to change. This underlines the dynamics of how the toilet market was created by regulation and how this affected the urban governance between government and business in toilet provision. Last, Chap. 6, "Concluding Remarks: A Moral-Capitalist Mode of Urban Governance of Public Toilets".

Notes

1. Hong Kong Government, 1899: 9.
2. Chadwick, 1882; Public Latrines in Hong Kong, *HKT*, 26 March 1891.
3. Chadwick, 1882: 18.
4. Chadwick, 1882: 20; Annual Medical Report for the Year 1931, *AR*, M44.
5. Cowell, 2003; Endacott, 1964; Yip, 2009.
6. Seat from Hong Kong Government, 1899: 7–10.
7. Anderson, 1995; Rogaski, 2006; Yeoh, 1996; Yu, 2010.
8. Anderson, 1995; Chadwick, 1882; Rogaski, 2006; Yeoh, 1996.
9. Harvey, 1982; Lefebvre, 1991; Logan and Molotch, 2007.
10. Melosi, 2005; Wohl, 1983.
11. Pierre, 2011:20; see also Pierre and Peters, 2000; Stone, 1993.
12. Shannon, 1989; So, 1986; Wallerstein, 2004.
13. So, 1986; Eng, 1986; Wong, 2017.
14. Guangdong Province Chorography, 2004: 275.
15. So, 1986: 80; Eng, 1986; Wong, 2017.
16. King, 1911; Ferguson, 2014; Xue, 2005; Yu, 2014.
17. Hong Kong Government, 1899: 6, 13.
18. CRN, HKRS149-2-534, 1869; Chadwick, 1882; Hong Kong Government, 1899.
19. Jackson, 2014; Melosi, 2005; Wohl, 1983; Yu, 2010.
20. For local economies, see Brunton, 2005; Jackson, 2014; Wohl, 1983. For regional economies, see King, 1911; Yeoh, 1996; Yu, 2010.
21. Douglas, 1970.
22. Laporte, 2000; Macpherson, 1987; Rogaski, 2004; Yu, 2010.
23. Chadwick, 1882.
24. HKRS38-2, *RB*, 1868–1930; Public Latrines in Hong Kong, *HKT*, 9 February and 26 March 1891.
25. CS/I001/00009951.GIF, Carl Smith Collection; Naturalization, *GG*, 11 July 1902, p. 1548.
26. Kwok himself, refers to Chap. 2. His son, see Naturalization, GG, 7 October 1899, p. 1555; CS/I003/00020641.GIF, Carl Smith Collection.
27. CS/I004/00035685.GIF, Carl Smith Collection.
28. CS/I004/00038035.GIF, Carl Smith Collection.
29. HKRS38-2, *RB*, 1870–1895.
30. Chadwick, 1882.
31. Population, *BB*, 1901, M2.
32. Water Closets in Hong Kong, *BB*, 1880.
33. CRN, HKRS149-2-534, 1869.
34. CRN, HKRS149-2, 1869–1887; Nightsoil Revenue, *BB*, 1890–1920; Revenue and Expenditure, *AR*, 1869–1930.
35. Hong Kong Government, 1899.
36. King, 1911; Prashad, 2001; Xue, 2005.

37. Disasters from Medical and Sanitary, *AR*, 1915 and 1916. Silk market from Eng, 1986; So, 1986. Landowners' action from, HKRS38-2, *RB*, 1900–1930.
38. Number from Hong Kong Government, 1899; HKRS38-2, *RB*, 1905, 1920, 1930.
39. Chadwick, 1882; Hong Kong Government, 1899.
40. Chadwick, 1842.
41. Bashford, 2005: 5.
42. Anderson, 1995; Andrews, 1996.
43. Douglas, 1970: 2.
44. Brunton, 2005; Freud, 1929.
45. Elias, 1978; Rogaski, 2004.
46. Glasco, 2010; Legg, 2007; Swanson, 1977.
47. Cowell, 2013; Munn, 2009; Pomfret, 2013.
48. Eitel, 1895: 192.
49. To the Editor of the Friend of China, *FoC*, 30 November 1843. Cowell, 2013.
50. Cowell, 2013; Evans, 1970; Munn, 2009.
51. Swanson, 1977.
52. Crowder, 1970; Curtin, 1964.
53. Andrews, 1996; Brunton, 2005.
54. Douglas, 1970; Elias, 1978.
55. Andrews, 1996; Barcan, 2010; Braverman, 2010; Brunton, 2005.
56. Foucault, 1980.
57. Brunton, 2005; Hamlin, 1998; Wright, 1960.
58. Driver, 1988; Legg, 2007; Yeoh, 1996.
59. Anderson, 1995; Rogaski, 2005; Yeoh, 1996.
60. Anderson, 1995.
61. *CSR*, *SP*, 1854; RCHK, Letter from Major-General to the Secretary for State for War, 5 February 1881. Enclosure in No. 34, *BPP* 1863–1881, Vol. 25, 1971, p. 708.
62. The mortality rate from Yellow Fever, *GG*, 12 May 1866, p. 189. The Parliament's concern from Observation by Surgeon General, 1 September 1880. Enclosure in No. 10, *BPP 1882–99*, Vol. 26, p. 37.
63. The Order and Cleanliness Ordinance, *GG*, 22 June 1867, No. 96, p. 232; CRN, HKRS149-2-534, 1869.
64. Chadwick, 1882.
65. Eitel, 1895; Endacott, 1964.
66. Hong Kong Government, 1887.
67. The population of the colony, CO129/51, 4 July 1855, p. 29.
68. Carroll, 2007; Tsai, 1993.
69. Abstract of the Net Revenue and Expenditure of Hong Kong, *BB*, 1878; Revenue and Expenditure, *BB*, 1879–1910.
70. Munn, 2009.
71. Chattopadhyay, 2005.
72. Dr. Ho Kai's Protest, *SP*, 27 May 1887, p. 404–7.
73. Gough Street Public Toilet, *SCMP*, 25 January 1906 and 18 January 1907.

74. Chu, 2013b; Scott, 1995.
75. Chadwick, 1882: 2, 42.
76. Chadwick, 1882; Hamilton, 1998.
77. Kidambi, 2007; Rogaski, 2005.
78. Bhabha, 1994.
79. Chadwick, 1882; Hong Kong Government, 1899.
80. Baverman 2010; Rogaski, 2005.
81. Foucault, 1980.
82. Ordinance for the Maintenance of Order and Cleanliness, *GG*, 22 June 1867, No. 96, p. 231–2; Instructions to Head Watchmen and Watchmen, *GG*, 23 June 1883, No. 223, p. 543–4.
83. HKRS38-2, *RB*, 1868–1920.
84. Tax from AJPH, *GG*, 11 February 1882, p. 82. Elite status from Carroll, 2007; Chan, 1991; Endacott, 1964; Sinn, 2003; Smith, 1971; Tsai, 1993.
85. Chu, 2013a; Endacott, 1964; Yip, 2009.
86. Carnoy, 1984; Miliband, 1973.
87. Thompson, 1983: 115–16.
88. Almond and Powell, 1978.
89. Carroll, 2007; Chan, 1991; Tsai, 1993; Sinn, 2003.
90. Chinese Houses, *GG*, 27 July 1878, p. 370–2.
91. Dr. Ho Kai's Protest, *SP*, 27 May 1887, p. 404–5.
92. Chu, 2013a; Endacott, 1964; Yip, 2009.
93. Carroll, 2007; Law, 2009; Sinn, 2003.
94. Lindblom, 1977.
95. HKRS38-2, *RB*, 1868–1895.
96. Foucault, 1978: 36.
97. Goodstadt, 2012.
98. Macpherson, 1996; Rogaski, 2004; Yu, 2010.

Chapter 2
Political-Economic Conditions for Chinese Business Elites Taking a Role in Governance

2.1 Overview

To consider why the colonial government and Chinese business elites partnered together in public toilet provision, we have to first examine the general political-economic conditions that enabled elites to take on a governance role in nineteenth century Hong Kong. It is necessary to delineate the salient features of colonial rule. First, the colony had to be self-financed, so it was undergoing a structural transformation towards land-centered capitalism. This opportunity quickly and enormously increased resources and wealth for the Chinese who could adapt to this new economic reality, increasing their capacity to participate in colonial governance. Second, regarding political aspects, to avoid conflict with the Chinese public, the government operated a strategy to distance itself from the daily life of society, which created a gap in the public services (e.g., education, medical, public health and social welfare) that were provided. Such racial tension was captured by the rising Chinese business elites. These factors meant that a rather different set of conditions developed, which brought out multilayered interactions between the government and the rising Chinese elites, ranging from economic collaboration in being partners in estate property development and commercial development, political collaboration by serving as intermediaries between the government and Chinese society, and social collaboration by providing public services and consulting on social affairs related to the colony. What lay behind elites intervening in colonial governance, which led to shared governance between them and the government? Was it a chance? Or did the government or Chinese create the situation? Who had control over the situation, or did no one have control?

This is not a detailed study of the rise of Chinese and colonial collaboration, and there have been many studies on these topics.[1] However, this analysis is concerned with analyzing the increasing public role of Chinese business elites in a new capitalist and colonial context that created the conditions for shared governance. By examining the political-economic conditions, the objective is to examine the context from which the elites intervened in colonial governance and to provide a dynamic account of elite

Y. Chong, *Toilet as Business for the Hygiene of the Chinese Community in Colonial Hong Kong*, https://doi.org/10.1007/978-981-19-1396-9_2

intervention in governance. The dynamics can be seen in two aspects: the vibrant economic restructuring that facilitated Chinese to accumulate wealth and resources. Second, the limitation of colonial rule created a gap between government and general Chinese, facilitating the intervenement of newly wealthy Chinese elites in colonial governance. These reflect how the colonial authority itself created the situation, and elites captured the opportunities for their own interest and Chinese as a whole.

In this chapter, the author first briefly discusses the Hong Kong colonial context wherein economic restructuring occurred and the rise of Chinese wealth and resource holdings set the stage for these newly risen Chinese business elites to help govern poor Chinese people. The second part focuses on how the limitations of colonial authority offered a gap for the extensive network of Chinese businessmen-based institutions crossed into social care, for example, TWH and the District Watch Force (DWF). These supported law and order and political-economic order, working to facilitate the entry of elites into colonial governance. Through these institutions, which were used as devices to capture the opportunities that arose in racial tensions, wealthy Chinese were able to act as spokesmen for their fellow countrymen, granting them tremendous political power and social capital. The third part covers these elites' entry into the formal political structure and their greater role in colonial policies. This analysis intends to develop a better understanding of elites' governance role, which is critical to their shared governance with the government of toilet provision.

2.2 Economic Restructuring: The Rise of Chinese Economic Capital and Land Resources

After the defeat of China to Britain in the First Opium War, Hong Kong officially made a colony in 1842; in the meantime, the British imperial government declared it a free port and made clear that this new colony had to be self-financing.[2] Not surprisingly, constrained by its free port inability to impose import duties, fiscal constraints were a top concern for the colonial government, particularly in the first four decades of its rule,[3] so it had to explore other sources of revenue. Lacking natural resources to sell, this situation freely led to the establishment of an opium monopoly, as there was a readymade opium market among the Mainland Chinese population. Economic constraints also encouraged the development of a land market. Here, the government not only aimed to generate revenue but also wanted to create an impression of permanency to attract wealthy Chinese to move to Hong Kong.[4] These two sources together amounted to approximately half of the total yearly government revenue through the nineteenth century.[5] This analysis focuses on the land market and explores how the institutionalization of a land market generated a new set of resources and power relations, including new government-business and colonizer-colonized relations. Chinese people within such a system became heavily involved because of the quick appreciation in the value of land, meaning that the strength of their land power, economic capital and tax paying ability greatly expanded. This strongly impacted the relationship between the government and Chinese and set the stage for the Chinese elites to take on a governance role. This section therefore first concerns where the land power and economic capital of these Chinese elites came from and then explores how this allowed them to enjoy a higher chance of gaining elite status, which facilitated their involvement in colonial governance.

2.2.1 *Chinese Heavy Land Investment and Increasing Tax Contribution*

It is interesting to note that soon after the British self-proclaimed sovereignty over Hong Kong, by 1841 (a year before Hong Kong was made officially made a colony), the first land sale had taken place.[6] Soon after the land market was established, there was a striking, nearly fourfold, increase in the property rate between 1845 and 1858, which accounted for approximately 25–45% of total yearly government revenue.[7] Between 1871 and 1877, land revenue became more consistent, accounting for between 3.2 and 15.2 percent of total revenue.[8] Land revenue grew from HK$208,827 to HK$895,067 between 1878 and 1910, a fourfold increase.[9] During this period, land revenue as a percentage of government revenue was approximately 10.7–31.3% (Fig. 2.1).

The rapidly growing land revenue was the result of acute competition for land from Chinese, beginning in the 1850s.[10] A large number of wealthy Chinese (e.g., Li Sing) hastened to invest in the land market when they emigrated from China to the colony, partly for the better economic opportunities offered in the colony, and partly to avoid the threat of the Taiping Rebellion (1850–64) in the Mainland. The land market with limited land supplies and an artificially elevated land price was such that the government and Chinese were both able to make huge profits. Operating within this

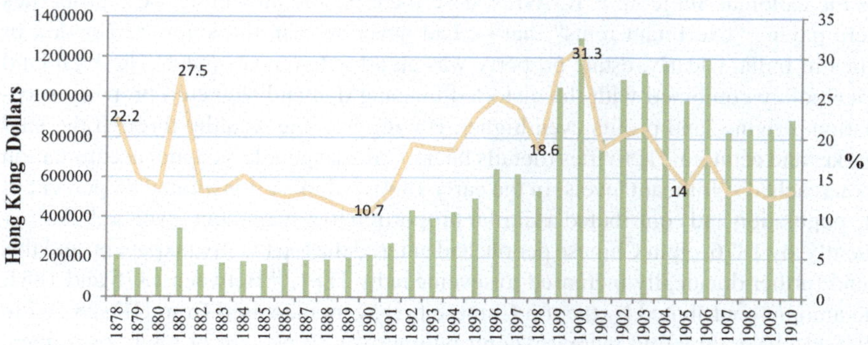

Fig. 2.1 Government land revenue and percentage of yearly revenue, 1878–1910. *Source* The author compiles and computes the percentage from abstract of the net revenue and expenditure of Hong Kong, *BB*, 1878; revenue and expenditure, *BB*, 1879–1910

scenario, the government delivered new opportunities to the most adaptable Chinese. As Carroll notes, "Colonialism in Hong Kong was not imposed upon a passive Chinese population. Nor did it involve slaughtering or driving out large numbers of indigenous peoples. Rather, colonialism attracted many merchants, contractors, and laborers from the mainland".[11] It is important to note, however, that some Chinese were in a position to benefit from colonialism,

Heavy Chinese investment in land went in parallel to the rising demand for housing, as the population kept increasing, especially of Chinese fleeing the Rebellion and trying their luck in the colony. The population grew from 39,017 in 1853 to 125,504 in 1865.[12] Throughout the three decades following the 1860s, the decade-average growth rate never dropped below 25%.[13] In the first fifty years of colonial rule, between 1841 and 1891, the population grew from 5,650 to 218,326,[14] generating tremendous opportunity for property investment. The investment was further driven by the concentrated population in the lower-western part (today Sheung Wan to Kennedy Town) of Victoria City. Chinese people were segregated to this area in 1844, as at the time they were considered to be the source of disease in the colony (discussed in Chap. 3). Ironically, this small area gradually became a "Chinatown" with vibrant commercial activities that attracted more fellow countrymen.[15] Therefore, the colony's already rapid population growth was concentrated in this area, which came to have nearly 65 percent (approximately 104,200 persons) of the Chinese living in the city by the late nineteenth century.[16]

The density of the ethnic enclave greatly distorted the demand and supply of housing, resulting in local housing shortages and price hikes. A great rise in land value always results in considerable increases in land revenue. Hong Kong's nascent property market attracted property speculators (both Chinese and European), who built low-cost, poor-quality tenement houses.[17] These houses achieved attractive returns. The houses were partitioned off, so a house with three rooms would be about fourteen square feet, with very small and basic kitchen attached, fetched from £55 to £70 a year. If it was a brothel, from £80 to £100 a year, in the 1870s.[18] As the Colonial Surgeon, P. B. Ayres, described, people inhabiting these properties were paying "exorbitant rents" that he had never seen in the slums of London or cities in India. Clearly, estate property was an attractive investment. The high land price policy combined with the distorted housing demand triggered property speculation, driving land profits even higher. Having become wealthy through the land market and economic activities (details later), Chinese people's capital accumulation soon reached significant levels. In the early 1860s, Chinese constituted 98 percent of the population and contributed a similar proportion to government revenue.[19] Subsequently, by 1876, eight Chinese people had entered the top twenty taxpayers, and this trend further drastically increased to seventeen by 1881.[20] Between 1876 and 1881, the amount contributed by the top Chinese taxpayers increased from HK$28,267 to HK$99,110, a threefold increase, contributing over 80 percent of total government revenue. The list of top taxpayers was a collection of Chinese elites, and as the author will show, some of them used their resources to have greater involvement in colonial governance.

The Chinese, especially landowners, contributed a considerable amount to government revenue and made the government deeply in favor of those invested in the land market, granting them a privileged position in the economic structure. Chinese people had been on the market since the 1840s,[21] but they were not allowed to purchase properties in European areas (today Admiralty and Central).[22] There was an emerging belief among the government that the Chinese were a threat to Europeans in physical and moral (racial degeneration) senses (will discuss in Chap. 3). By managing the "disease contagion" of Chinese, a clause in building leases specified lessees should not erect houses that did not conform in character to others in the neighborhood, this restricted Chinese houses, which were small and overcrowded and so would be considered insanitary, from being built in European areas.[23] The situation was changed in 1878. In the name of justice, Governor Hennessy (1877–82) argued that the Chinese tax contribution and commercial activities were key to economic prosperity and recommended that the British government relax the restriction.[24]

With Hennessy's support, Chinese were finally allowed to purchase properties and build Chinese houses in European areas, giving them a large new opportunity to accumulate land and quick returns on their investments. There were two main factors driving Hennessy to support this decision. First was the growing proportion of taxes contributed by the Chinese, as noted. Second was the cutting down of European firms due to Chinese competition, which could market European goods and supply Chinese goods from the Mainland to Europe more cheaply.[25] The spread of Chinese shops accelerated and required more urban space for commercial development. The relaxation meant Chinese were no longer confined to set areas (the lower-western part of Victoria City), which was met with strong opposition from the military and government officials, who both perceived Chinese as possessing pathological bodies because of their insanitary hygiene behavior (open defecation) and living style (crowded living), which most affected the health of the troops (will discuss the details in Chap. 3).[26] Hennessy was criticized as being deeply attached to the Chinese to the point that he compromised public health in return for better relations, particularly as the Chinese landed class was a major source of revenue.[27] Prevailing over the dissenting views, he approved a partial lift of the building restrictions that allowed only Europeans to sell houses and building sites to Chinese below Caine Road and Wyndham Street in Central.[28] This was due to the belief that altitude affected the circulation of fresh air, which was significant to drive away miasma.[29]

There were three other results from the relaxation of how Chinese used urban space: first was that the Chinese greatly expanded their land ownership, second was the worries of higher chance of disease transmission of Chinese leading to Chadwick's investigation of Hong Kong sanitary condition, and third was the enactment of the European District Reservation Ordinance further segregated Chinese and Europeans (more details in Chap. 3). Despite opposition from military and government officials to the relaxation between 1879 and 1881, there was a remarkable transfer of property from European to Chinese hands. The total value of property bought by Chinese people from Europeans or the government amounted to HK$1,710,036 and HK$17,705, respectively.[30] In contrast, the value bought by Europeans from Chinese or the government was much lower, just HK$16,450 and HK$5,060, respectively.

Chinese entered a new period of rapid growth in wealth and land resources, and this enormous land transfer implied a potential shift of urban space from European to Chinese control and the increasing tax contribution of Chinese, as noted earlier. It is said that the tax of Chinese rose radically due to the 1881 property rush, triggered by Chinese property speculators.[31] Leaving aside the question of the property rush, it is apparent that the colony's economic growth had long relied on Chinese investment, which outnumbered that of foreigners' tax contributions, which fell from HK$62,523 to HK$21,032, a reduction of 200 percent. High land control had a significant influence on political and economic aspects and significantly influenced the distribution of elite statuses, which was characterized by their landownership.[32]

2.2.2 Chinese Land Ownership and Elite Status

Chinese wealth and land holdings greatly increased, meaning they formed not only an economic pillar that supplied a critical boost to government revenue but also controlled the critical resource, land, that could reshape the usage of urban space. This consolidated their fundamental structural position in the economic system. It seems almost too obvious that Governor Hennessy would favor Chinese, especially the landed class, which could pay large amounts of tax. Especially at a time when growth in government revenue was primarily based on property investment. In an address to the Legislative Council, Hennessy highly recognized the contribution of Chinese taxpayers: "as long as they desire to establish themselves and their descendants in the colony forever, so long we have a guarantee for loyalty and good order."[33] This made the government respect Chinese voices, forming the backbone of a new state of relations between the government and Chinese.[34] It is interesting to see what distinctive set of socioeconomic and political relations emerged in the structural transformation of the economic system based upon land-centered capitalism, which eventually led to the government treating landed-based Chinese as elites.

The formation of a status group based on owning land resources was not a coincidence; rather, the social environment (e.g., the level of commercialization) and resources available decide the type of elite in different areas.[35] This echoes Parkin's argument that aristocrat elites with blue blood in a feudal society were replaced by business elites with wealth in nineteenth century European industrial society.[36] Central to this replacement is the emerging industrial order, which was based upon banking, commerce, trade, and professional qualifications. Parkin argues that a hierarchy of economic class rather than royalty is the truth behind the distribution of elite status in the modern world. Although elite status is not necessarily synonymous with wealth, it does have a positive correlation. He emphasizes that status is a valuable, unevenly distributed resource, which underlines a common situation, where some groups are better placed than others to gain status. That the status distribution highly correlates to the hierarchy of economic class that lies in the stratifications of occupation based upon the functional importance (managers over factory workers in terms of greater contribution to the production output) or skills (manual and professional jobs over unskilled and semiprofessional jobs) and that an important feature of this stratification is deeply rooted in the degree of skill scarcity in the market. Moreover, people from a higher occupation order are more likely to enjoy higher wages and own property, meaning they could accumulate wealth and enjoy a higher chance of gaining status.

The same was true in capitalist Hong Kong in the nineteenth century. When the colonial government, embedded in land capitalist logic with rapid and sustainable urbanization, was commonly adopted in economic restructuring, land was undoubtedly the principal source of government revenue. This profoundly changed the way the government approached Chinese people, privileging those who were invested in the land market, earning them an elite status, and creating a land-based Chinese class. This is particularly significant when land resources, significantly controlled by Chinese, had structural importance in the economic and political spheres. Smith noted that "the relation of land ownership to elite status can be judged by a list of the twenty highest rate payers in 1876 and 1881".[37] This indicates that those qualifying as elites by virtue of economic importance were those controlling huge land holdings, and they came to be a significant contributor to government revenue. The business class, socially the lowest, being wealthy through land investment became elites. This elite group was very different from the elites of the traditional Chinese status hierarchy. Traditional elites' status originated from being a member of the gentry (attained from civil service examination) to farmers, laborers and businessmen.[38] As far as early colonial Hong Kong, a hierarchy of economic class, in terms of paying tax and land resource possession, was fundamental to the distributive mechanisms of elite status, wherein the middle and professional classes were not well established.[39] Elite status, in terms of land ownership, was therefore a way to conceptualize Chinese's political and economic importance.

In addition to enjoying high land prices and huge demand, Chinese businesses extended their business to other fields rapidly and increased their commercial activities. There were many opportunities, as the colony's port role was rapidly growing from the increasing trade catering to Chinese emigrants and indentured laborers in Australia, the Straits, and the United States.[40] The following vibrant activities help to drive prosperity from commercial activities. In 1871 and 1881, the number of businessmen increased from 2,144 to 6,885, including a sharp rise in the number of bankers from zero to 55, compradors from 76 to 95, and traders from 65 to 2,377.[41] Trade between local businesses and countries across the world blossomed too, including Britain, China, India and Southeast Asia.[42] There was a wide array of commodities, cotton, tea, shark fins, to timber, including notorious trade items such as opium and coolies. Comparing the business of British businessmen in Hong Kong and West Indian Islands, Hennessy attributed the success in Hong Kong to the national character of Chinese who were "a community industrious and temperate, with a natural aptitude for commerce".[43] He highly acknowledged the vital role that Chinese played in developing the colony's prosperity, reflecting his willingness to accord esteem and deference to them.

Growing wealth through the land market and commercial activities could be converted into higher social status, so here, the government's relationship towards

Chinese being so strongly influenced by the tax they paid epitomizes the significant effect of economic restructuring on colonial rule.[44] A distinctive set of new power relations gradually emerged between the colonial government and Chinese business elites, whose growing economic capital and social status allowed them a privileged voice in colonial governance, meaning a pattern of colonial collaboration centered on shared governance was formed, allowing Chinese to play a greater role in the daily operation of the colony.

2.3 Chinese Elites Intervening in Colonial Governance

Colonialism rooted in capitalism attracted a large number of Mainland Chinese to Hong Kong. This also generated new problems of urban life, such as disease, pauperism, and petty crime, which required public services for the capitalist system and colonial rule to continue to function and be sustainable, benefitting both the colonial government and Chinese elites. However, the government had a limited capacity (manpower and revenue) and lacked interest in providing such services to the general Chinese population. Playing into the above anxieties and the pressing need to maintain law and order and provide welfare and sanitation, the government encouraged these elites, who, in assuming a high moral position and responsibility for the well-being of Chinese society, moved to help provide public services and govern poor Chinese people. The making of colonial collaboration between government and elites was not separated from the limitations of colonial rule. This is explained well by Ronald Robinson,

> The amount of force at the disposal of colonial rulers locally seemed tiny in comparison with the possibility of disaffection and revolt. Reinforcement was usually sent with reluctance, the need for it regarded as a sign of administrative incompetence. Coercion was expensive and counterproductive except in emergencies, and everyone knew that no amount of force could hold down indigenous politics for a long time.[45]

Undoubtedly, the amount of force and financial support disbursed by the government was far from sufficient to sustain its rule, so there was a pressing need for effective governance. Considering that underlying racial tensions might arise in managing Chinese people's customs (ancestor worship, keeping concubines and maid child servant) and lifestyles (sanitary behavior and way of living), the government promised Chinese that they would be governed in accordance with their own customs and laws.[46] Therefore, the colonial relationship was further shaped by a strategy of "boundary consciousness".[47] Colonial governments played an important role in preserving structures of racial segregation. A general argument was that the political characteristics of colonial rule—the notion of "boundary consciousness", coined by Lau—explains the government's reluctance to take up its public role to provide public services for the Chinese.[48] The gist of the argument is that cries of minimal intervention from colonial bureaucrats, that the government is better to distance itself from Chinese customs and daily lives to avoid racial tensions. As a consequence of a segregated colonial relationship, Lau argues that "the bureaucracy does not pursue 'state activism' nor intrude unnecessarily into society to restructure it, and it is successful both in depoliticizing society and in resolving the residual and outstanding societal problems left unsolved by society".[49] This offered a basis for the government to be detached from societal issues.

2.3.1 *Securing Revenue and Colonial Operation with the Help of Chinese Elites*

This style of colonial rule was characterized by "boundary consciousness", creating a gap for public service provision to the Chinese community, which was filled by Chinese elites and their social organizations. Clearly, maintaining law and order and offering services to the community were largely handled by elites. Sinn is correct to note that "these functions were all the more necessary since the Hong Kong government was for the most part unable or unwilling to perform them".[50] This finally led the government to offer opportunities to the elites to augment their pieces of public power. Desiring to secure revenue without the government intervening in Chinese daily life and causing racial conflict, the government adopted the farming system by auctioning out resources such as opium, stone and night soil, in which it had exercised a controlling interest. The farming system worked where the successful bidders (called farmers) had to pay the government a yearly rental for the monopoly of controlling the resource or service. Such systems were widely employed in Asian colonies and concessions, such as Singapore, Shanghai and Tianjin, under foreign administration.[51] In Hong Kong, dispensing monopolies achieved 10 to 25 percent of yearly government revenue between the 1840s and 1870s.[52] However, the farming system was more than economic collaboration, it also achieved political goals by using Chinese to provide public services (e.g., night soil collection) to Chinese and control Chinese farmers in their practical operation, and so avoid racial conflicts (intervening in Chinese daily life and practices) while securing revenue. Munn unravels the underlying political calculation of the government,

> By auctioning off revenue collection rights to middlemen, the government was able to secure an income with minimal trouble and liability: it was relieved of much of bother and friction of collecting tax direct from the people; it was assured of an income, since the rental was payable monthly in advance and the farmers were heavily bonded; and it could distance itself from the farms if things went wrong. The farms also had a political value…intended 'as a mere assertion of sovereignty', to drive out revenue collectors from the Chinese government…In policing their revenue, farmers also contributed to the general preservation of order in the colony.[53]

Apart from wealth accumulation, the government also relied on the farmers for advice relating to the operation of the system, signaling their involvement in colonial governance.[54] The Governor J. Davis wrote:

> A system of collection that of all others is the best adapted to a Chinese population. As the farmers themselves are Chinese, their perfect knowledge of their own country-men joined to

the personal interest that they have in the collection, rendering them incomparably the best tax-gatherers in a case of this kind.[55]

The farming system's advantages were mutual, which also contributed to the possibility of wealth accumulation and the opportunity to build political influence and power for the farmers. The increasing wealth of Wo Hang Opium Firm, which was owned by Li Sing and his nephews such as Li Tak Cheong, is a good example.[56] Since Li Sing came to Hong Kong in the early 1850s, he heavily invested in land and tendered for the opium monopoly through the firm during the 1870s and 1880s.[57] This was a major factor contributing to Wo Hang becoming the twelfth top taxpayer in 1876, further rising to the first in 1881, contributing HK$11,397.[58] Li Sing himself was the eleventh in 1876, and when he died in 1900, he left over HK$ 6 million, a huge amount at the time.[59] Meanwhile, Li Tak Cheong foundered Lai Hing Hong (an opium firm), which was granted the opium monopoly between 1873 and 1876.[60] The firm was one of the first three Chinese firms elected to be members of the Hong Kong General Chamber of Commerce in 1880; the Chamber had the power to nominate an unofficial Legislative Councilor.[61] The two other firms were Sun Yee Hong and Tak On Bank. This was seen as a recognition of the growing importance of Chinese business by their European counterparts.[62] Other non-Chinese members included Opium dealer E.R. Bellios, the renowned real estate merchant H.N. Mody, and W. Keswick of Jardine Matheson & Co. Having become wealthy through land investment and opium, Li Sing and Li Tak Cheong became heavily involved in the social sphere of Hong Kong society; the former was the founding director of TWH, while the latter was the director in the 1870s,[63] and they were both appointed as members of the Committee on Emigration of Women to US in the mid-1870s, for example.[64] Indeed, the farming system delivered "the possibility of great wealth" to Chinese that we will see the night soil farming system was widely employed in Hong Kong in Chap. 3.

2.3.2 *Involvement in Colonial Governance Through Institutions*

As wealth and land were increasingly concentrated in the hands of a minority of Chinese from the 1860s, this signified a rise of economic capital, and Chinese economic elites became confident enough to increase their involvement in colonial governance through establishing and engaging in philanthropic institutions and social organizations. While the limitations of colonial rule over a foreign population created a gap in responding to the challenges posed by Chinese, colonial relationships facilitated the social and political rise of Chinese elites and their organizations. As more services were provided by the organizations instead of the government, the elites' influence on the Chinese populace increased.

Traditionally, Chinese elites entered the social sphere after having established themselves in business. This does not mean they were not altruistic. In terms of

Chinese culture, the Chinese phrase "virtue comes after wealth" best describes the rationale behind elites' active involvement in social issues. Through displays of virtue, they sought to assume a high moral position, building up their social status. In the early stages of colonization, compradors, contractors, civil servants and landowners were perceived as elites, who wanted to show that they were the responsible class in terms of maintaining law and order and caring for the welfare of the local society, rather than being seen as sojourners or profit hunters.[65] For example, in 1859, a newly risen elite Tang Luk contributed to a school book fund for Chinese students attending government schools when he became a main stone-quarry contractor.[66] Tang rose from a humble background, starting his career as a stone cutter in the 1850s, family legend claims that he earned "the first pot of gold" from the construction of Pokfulam reservoir and Tai Tam reservoir.[67] Nevertheless, no documentary proof of his connection with the two reservoirs has been found, but one point to be sure of is he climbed up the social ladder and became the main stone-quarry contractor in Hong Kong, founding Yuen Cheong Hong, a leading stone quarry company.[68] Tang was also a significant landowner who owned at least seventy pieces of land by 1880, and he was the twelfth top taxpayer in 1881.[69] At his death in 1887, he left a considerable estate of HK$208,699.[70]

From the 1850s, one feature of Chinese elites' involvement in colonial governance was a gradual movement from engaging on an individual basis to an institutional basis, through which the elites guided the colony's development by forming social institutions that still exist today, such as Po Leung Kuk (PLK), TWH, and Nam Pak Hong.[71] These well-established networks of businessmen-controlled institutions were formulated by Chinese business elites, who were compradors, merchants and top taxpayers (mainly landowners). The unique arrangement of the business elites in this respect was chiefly due to two factors. First, the elites sought to build up their social status by holding a director position and providing public services to the general Chinese population. The business class held low status in feudal Chinese society; therefore, possessing high social status was the ultimate means of bringing pride and honor to one's family and ancestors for traditional Chinese. This represented an understanding that what was being measured was the social worth of these institutions and knowing the personal social status to be gained from holding a director position.[72] This is particularly true for being members of DWF or directors of TWH, which were highly honored by the government for their service and help in maintaining peace for the colony.

Second, the elites' concern with economic prosperity and social stability was another major factor coloring the establishment of the social organizations, which were social care organizations and a town watch operating as a local police force. Their presence tilted towards governance towards a mode shared between them and the government.[73] It was the emergence of capitalist development that created the conditions for the self-interest of elites, inducing them to act as active social agents in providing public services to their fellow countrymen and maintaining law and order, which were important requirements for prosperous development. It was the urban/capitalist social structure that created this opportunity to invest economic capital into acquiring political capital, an opportunity that did not exist in Mainland

China, as the political system was largely still feudal. Through the provision of public services and maintaining public order, these social organizations provided an avenue for elites to affect the everyday realities of colonial governance in a proactive manner. At the beginning of colonization in the nineteenth century, these organizations were particularly important for suppressing crime, providing services, mediating social disputes among Chinese, and settling riots and strikes to maintain political and social stability.

In the highly segregated Hong Kong society of early colonial rule, social and political instabilities stemming from lower-class Chinese were serious concerns for the government. Midgal notes that the involvement of local elites in colonial governance was at the time seen by colonial governments as a means of ensuring security and stability for its rule; therefore, they carefully chose elites who were resourceful, wealthy and influential in the local community.[74] This ultimately obliged the Hong Kong colonial government to give the Chinese elites and their organizations tremendous new authority (e.g., patrolling the Chinese community with their own police force and possessing magistracy power over social disputes among Chinese), enabling them to establish a hierarchy of power facilitating the cultivation of social influence over the Chinese community.[75] This obviously created privileged access for some elites, such as Kwok Acheong and Ho Kai, and organizations such as DWF and TWH, that were preferred by the government and had influential effects on colonial governance.[76] As Lethbridge describes the network of Chinese social organizations as a system of "prestige, influence and power, a hierarchical one".[77] Here, the author will talk about the police force, DWF, and the colony's most prominent Chinese social organization, TWH, as the main institutionalization of Chinese power in the late nineteenth century, which shows how Chinese elites formed these institutions to take social positions and what made the government share power with them, facilitating their intervention in colonial governance.

Both Chinese and European businessmen formed their own civil corps from the 1850s due to the corrupt and drunken police force (mainly comprised of Indians and discharged European sailors) that was unable to control crime to protect their commercial interests.[78] However, Kaifong leaders, who were prominent merchants and shopkeepers of the Chinese quarter, continued to propose a self-policing system to the government. This was in vain until 1866, when it was rumoured that lower-class Chinese from Guangdong were planning to loot and burn houses of Chinese elites. These elites soon made use of this fear and lobbied the government to allow them to legalize their civil corps into district watchmen, an action that formed the DWF.[79] From the British point of view, lower class Chinese were basically criminals who would deter the more respectable Chinese from moving to or staying in the colony, endangering economic development.[80] Considering that watchmen were completely funded by Chinese but assisted the government in maintaining law and order under the supervision of the Registrar General, Governor R. G. MacDonnell (1865–72) was certainly happy to endorse the plan. However, Chinese people having their own police force meant that the government had to forego complete control over the Chinese population and allow Chinese elites to intervene in public order, which had far-reaching consequences for their own goals to seize pieces of public power and status.

In Lethbridge's words, Kaifong associations (neighborhood associations) were "simply groups of civic-minded, status-seeking, and paternalistic citizens in a particular area of the city who set themselves up, [and] voted themselves in as a public body" to engage in the public sphere.[81] Kaifong leaders were self-proclaimed leaders, and the elections were just a ritual to legitimize power among the Chinese community. They collected funds from businessmen and paid the watchmen, who had policing power as police constables and were then appointed by the Governor on the recommendation of the kaifong.[82] Holding police powers and being well known to the inhabitants of their district, by the 1880s the duties of the watchmen had extended to assisting the government to conduct censuses, working with the sanitary inspectors to supervise the daily operation of public toilets and night soil removal, and helping the PLK to detect human trafficking by rescuing kidnapped children and women who were at risk of exploitation.[83]

In 1891, the Force was transformed into the District Watch Committee, which was coopted into the government administration system, meaning that watchmen were included in the Civil Service List and paid out of public funds.[84] Of the twelve members of the first committee, ten were directors or ex-directors of PLK or TWH, the two early influential Chinese social organizations. The two most prominent members were definitely Ho Kai and Wei Yuk. It is true that such an official connection with the government helped smooth the flow of favor from the general Chinese population to the government and vice versa, a privilege unmatched by other organizations.[85] It was the Committee, which Mills describes as the "Chinese Executive Council of Hong Kong", which developed into one of the most influential political bodies.[86] In a sense, this allowed the Chinese to govern themselves. The government consulted the Committee on various issues related to the daily operation of the colony, ranging from the regulation of Chinese theatres to the appointment of midwives. In addition, the Committee helped to maintain political stability, for example, by mediating the strike-boycott of 1925–26.[87]

Similarly, the original purpose of the establishment of TWH was that the government was unable to offer proper and free medical services (vaccination and outpatient clinic service) for poor Chinese individuals. In practice, TWH did not restrict itself to delivering such services; it also housed the poor, offered free education, sent human remains back to China to be buried, and cared for kidnapped children and women, for example.[88] Another important organization, PLK, was created to protect vulnerable women and children to maintain social stability, an important requirement for prosperous development.[89] TWH not only provided much of the needed services to the Chinese community but also helped the organization manage public affairs by arbitrating civil and commercial disputes among Chinese people. Culturally, Chinese considered that going to court would bring bad luck and so would avoid it whenever possible. This was particularly true in a colonial context with an alien legal system. Therefore, TWH served as a tribunal to mediate or settle disputes among Chinese, which included creditors claiming repayment from debtors or craftsman whose apprentices had run away. This helped resolve disputes, keeping peace and order in the colony.

Moreover, much evidence also shows that TWH worked with the government to settle political conflicts, such as the 1872 cargo workers' strike and the 1884 anti-French riot, all involving large numbers of lower-class Chinese.[90] The main reason behind its involvement in these conflicts was that political and social stability was seen to be crucial to economic development, which motivated the directors (all businessmen) to collaborate with the government to settle the crises.[91] Certainly, Chinese people were divided by class when public and private interests conflicted, as we will see more in the next chapter. The reason for TWH's success in the arbitration of conflicts was that the government relied heavily on it to provide services to Chinese society, allowing it to use its highly prized social capital as a basis for exerting socio-political influence on the public, for example urging strikers to return to work.[92] Tsai argues that such capital was built upon a mix of "wealth, moral authority, and prestige", consisting of a combination of economic capital, moral commitments to provide welfare to their fellow countrymen, and recognition by the colonial government.[93]

Through the networks of social organizations, the elites took advantage of the racial segregation that existed between the government and local society, presenting themselves as social leaders of Chinese society but also actually reinforcing the segregation. The interdependence between the government and elites was strengthened in parallel to the segregation so that the elites played an important social role in this segregated society, which made the government recognize their power between it and general society.[94] This set the stage for the elites' greater involvement in colonial governance and was conducive to making them a partner of the government. The growing sociopolitical influence of Chinese elites, who took key positions in social organizations, became strong enough to become involved in different aspects of colonial governance. Rather than simply being dichotomous or collaborative, the relationship between the government and Chinese elites in reality was more complex. Their involvement in wide-ranging public services, even law and order, obligated the government to join with the elites as strategic partners, absorbing them into the political sphere. More importantly, this allowed elites to maintain a particular position in the colony and consequently brought about gaining formal political appointments.

2.4 An Entry into Political Circles

Thus far, we have seen how Chinese elites acquired significant economic and social capital in Hong Kong. This raises the question of how the economic and social capital of Chinese elites allows them to enter the formal political structure and intervene in colonial decision-making processes.

2.4.1 A Recognition of Chinese Economic Contributions

Sinn argues that the directors of social organizations contributed to economic development and political crisis settlement through philanthropic works and public services, which would earn them either an elite status or a political appointment, and so is best understood as a convergence of power and charity.[95] These efforts made the government publicly honor donors and their social organizations. This is best marked by the high-profile ceremonial visit to TWH by Hennessy in February 1878, the first instance of a governor making a formal visit to a Chinese organization. This high-profile political gesture signified a recognition of Chinese contributions. The government gazette detailed the grand occasion,

> Approximately 2:30 P.M. a guard of honour from the 74th Regiment, with the Regimental Band, arrived, and lined the road leading to the Hospital…The Chinese community was very fully represented, there being present nearly 300 influential local residents from all classes of the community; and of those present some 50 or 60 were in their Mandarin costumes, some with blue buttons, some with crystal, and some with gold buttons, while a few had the additional honor of wearing the peacock's feather…as the Governor and party entered, a salute of three guns was fired and some Chinese music was performed.[96]

Public interest was in the ceremonial expression of both British government and Chinese elites, particularly those wearing Mandarin outfits, which were modelled on those worn by high-ranking Chinese officials in the Qing dynasty (1636–1912). Official Chinese titles could be purchased from the Chinese government from the 1850s onwards due to the fiscal deficit in the royal coffers suffering from the Taiping Rebellion.[97] The significance of expression was as Tobin argues, "displaying oneself dressed in another culture's clothing can be a form of empowerment as well as appropriation".[98] This was particularly important in early colonization as the hierarchy of traditional Chinese culture was reinforced by this expression so that the elites were probably literally endowed with magisterial power within the Chinese community, which helped the government solve minor conflicts.[99] Equally important to note is that among those in the outfits at the event were a number of large landowners and top taxpayers, including Kwok Acheong, Cheng Sing Yeong and Ng Sang (all three of them were also toilet landowners, more details in alter chapters). Kwok Acheong was among the very few Tanka to rise to prominence; he later became a comprador to the Peninsular and Oriental Steam Navigator Company (P & O Co), a post he held for many years from the mid-1840s.[100]

As a socially disadvantaged group, Tanka were boat people who had long been discriminated against by land-dwelling people. This was because Tanka could not own land and had no established gentry. They were prohibited from taking the civil service examination, the main way to enter the gentry elite.[101] Even though the prohibition was lifted by Emperor Yong Zheng (reigned 1678–1735) of the Ching dynasty in the early 1700s,[102] Tanka still struggled to create gentry and continued to be discriminated against, leading to their unequal position in society. From this disadvantaged position, Tanka was active on the waterways of the Pearl River Delta (near Hong Kong), meaning they easily established contact with foreign businessmen, who were largely confined to the Chinese coastline by the Chinese government. This was conducive to the collaboration between Tanka and the British. Kwok started his legendary relationship with Great Britain when he piloted the HMS Nemesis during the capture of the Bogue Fort in Canton in the First Opium War.[103] He also supplied the British Navy with provisions when it was engaged with Chinese forces.

Working with the British was a sure way to climb the social ladder, especially for discriminated people such as Kwok Acheong. Eventually, he was famed for his services to the British during the war, which gave him the opportunity to accumulate wealth, prestige and power when Hong Kong was established afterwards. Kwok was first a comprador to the P & O Co. and became one of the founders of the European-owned Hong Kong, Canton and Macao Steamboat Company in 1865 (he later retired from the board of directors at the end of 1868).[104] Later, with shipwright William Bolton Spratt, he started his own steamship company, Cosmopolitan Dock Co., in the 1870s and became the owner of thirteen steamers, including the German steamer *Olympia*, purchased for about HK$90,000.[105] A strong steamship allowed him to compete with the Hong Kong, Canton and Macao Steamboat Company, and Kwok became the first “Chinese shipping tycoon”. His other businesses included bakeries and a monopoly of cattle imports, which earned him the nickname of “Ngau Lan Atsung” (Cattle Market Atsung).[106]

In 1876, he was the third top taxpayer. He was one of the elites wearing a peacock’s feather. at the ceremonial visit of Governor Hennessy to Tung Wah Hospital in 1878.[107] Furthermore, he was also commonly consulted by Hennessy on local issues and accompanied the governor on visits to factories.[108] However, his ascension was high-risk, and Kwok Acheong’s son was detained by the Chinese authorities in 1878 as punishment for his betrayal in Anglo-Chinese conflicts. Due to Kwok’s great contributions, the British Consul mediated the dispute, and his son was eventually released. When he died in 1880, prominent among those paying public tribute to him were representatives of the Governor and the Military Department, the Colonial Secretary and the Chinese Secretary. His funeral procession was described as being of “remarkable grand proportions, and the elaborate and costly paraphernalia with which it was adorned showed that no expense had been spared in getting it up”.[109] Such an enormous procession ran from his home at Queen’s Road West to Kennedy Town and took more than one hour to pass one spot. It was a fitting end to Kwok’s legendary rise.

Seeing war collaborators like Kwok Acheong be rewarded for their service to the British and being transformed into new elites compelled more adaptable Chinese to act as middleman between Chinese and Europeans in trade and social issues. Colonial collaborators were certainly incentivized with rewards, and the government granted them land and monopolies (mainly opium and stone), which were two important sources of long-term significant wealth. This contributed to the domestic rise of certain Chinese people, as Carroll remarks, “By rewarding such men with privileges—for example, land grants—and offering them lucrative monopolies, the government helped foster the growth of a local Chinese gentry”.[110] Law moves a step further and adds that “Collaboration with the Westerners brought to them not only economic gain but also advancement in political and social status".[111] The advancement of individuals impacted Chinese as a whole, as the Chinese elites were appointed to different advisory committees and appointed as unofficial Legislative Councilors, Sanitary Board members, or JPs who could nominate unofficial Legislative Councilors. These appointments represent the Chinese elites' growing and increasingly formal relationship with the government; this relationship will be analyzed further.

Next is Ching Sing Yeong, the ninth top taxpayer in 1881, who was a partner to Hong Kong Fire Insurance Co. (founded by Jardine Matheson & Co.) and founder of Tak On Bank; which as shown, was one of the Chinese firms to join the Hong Kong General Chamber of Commerce in 1880. Additionally, Ng Sang ranked ninth in 1876 but rapidly rose to second in 1881 as his tax contribution increased from HK$2,570 to HK$10,240.[112] He was comprador to Douglas Lapraik & Co., a large British-owned shipping company, and a partner of Wong Li Cheng Hong, which exported Chinese silk and tea to Britain.[113] His business achievements attracted the government's attention, and he was appointed as a member of the Committee on Emigration of Women to the United States in the mid-1870s.[114] However, Ng Sang was not that lucky, and he suffered huge losses in the 1881 property mania, which was said to be an immediate cause of his death. According to Smith, Ng "fell victim to the fever of land speculation in 1881 and suffered heavy losses. Concern over his strained financial position so affected his health that he died in 1883. Action was brought by his employers against the Ng family property to cover debts he left".[115]

After examining the visit of Governor Hennessy to TWH and the prominent Chinese elites who greeted the governor that day, we now turn attention to the practical effect of the elites' economic and social capital. This is reflected in a memorial petition of seventy-two Chinese individuals and institutions, including TWH, who supported Li Tak Cheong's original building plan by opposing the health-based requirement for additional ventilation in tenement houses made by the Surveyor General.[116] In response to the government's building proposal, the memorialists presented themselves as spokesmen for the Chinese community and argued that lower-class Chinese were culturally accustomed to overcrowding and closed the windows for security reasons, so it was unnecessary to provide more air or light. With the prestigious memorialists, Hennessy cautioned his subordinates that the memorial was signed by "intelligent and influential Chinese residents whose views with respect to such questions are entailed to the greatest weight", it was thus a certainty that the proposal for additional ventilation would be shelved.[117]

It is not an exaggeration to say the memorial was signed by all the Chinese elites, as owning land was a very important and common feature to elite wealth, showing how a small group could be mobilized by collective interests. This group included important people such as Ching Sing Yeong, Kwok Acheong, Li Sing, Ng Sang, Tang Luk, Ip Chuk Kai (comprador to Reiss & Company, partner of Sun On Bank and ex-director of TWH),[118] Leong On (comprador to Gibbs, Livingston & Company, partner of Sun On Bank and founding director of TWH),[119] and three future Legislative Councilors: Ho Kai, Wei Yuk and Wong Shing. There was an interlocking relationship between the landowning memorialists and a number of key parties: compradors, top taxpayers and the directors of TWH. Of the seventy-two memorialists, 10 percent were compradors, and 11 percent were top taxpayers and directors (present and past) of TWH.[120] TWH, which owned sixteen houses, also signed the memorial.[121] Property investment was a way to accumulate funds, which was important for it to support all types of public services for the Chinese community that could not be obtained through government subsidies.[122]

By focusing on the economic and social capital of Chinese elites, we have seen how these accumulations of capital were regarded highly by the government. In the following, we will see how that capital was translated into political power. In doing so, this made the government bring the elites into the formal political structure, allowing them to play a greater role in colonial governance.

2.4.2 Political Appointments: Chinese Enter the Political Circle

The Legislative Council and the Executive Council were the two top government organs in the colonial era, through which Chinese people participated in the policy-making and management of public affairs, safeguarding their interests (e.g., economic interests, habits and customs). At the same time, these appointments avoided or lessened Chinese opposition to the government. For the government, the ability of Chinese to flourish in business was of great interest and made Hennessy accept the Chinese elites' suggestion of appointing a Chinese Councilor. Hennessy made it clear that it was time to have Chinese representation on the Council when he said,

> I was justified in recommending the Queen to appoint a Chinese member on the Legislative Council in a Colony where so much of the commercial life is conducted by Chinese; where the wealthiest merchants are Chinese, where the Chinese possess so much property, where they are the permanent inhabitants, and where nine-tenths of the government revenues are contributed by them.[123]

Under the support of Hennessy, in 1878 and 1880, the two most honorable political appointments were probably the first Chinese JP and the first Legislative Councilor, given to Ng Choy, known as Wu Ting Fang, who was educated in Britain and became the first Chinese barrister practicing in Hong Kong.[124] Ng was the founding director of TWH, and one of the representatives dressed in Mandarin outfits, in which he gave a welcome speech during Hennessy's visit to TWH in 1878.[125] According to Smith, the original favorite candidate for the appointment of Councilor was Leong On, who in return recommended Ng Choy as he was educated in the West and so might be equipped with a wider viewpoint and so could better represent Chinese interests.[126] However, Ng himself was also involved in the land market,[127] although he was not a major landowner or businessmen; nonetheless, this shows that his appointment was not made purely on personal grounds. It was evident that economic and social considerations entered into the decision, reflecting the economic and social importance of Chinese.

It is evident that economic and social considerations entered into the decision, reflecting the economic and social importance of Chinese people who received the appointment. Sinn describes the appointment as "a landmark in the history of the Chinese community, giving it a new sense of importance" and a departure from the segregation policy adopted in the first four decades of colonial rule.[128] Nonetheless, we should not overestimate the importance of the appointments, after all the two Councils (Executive Council and Legislative Council) were established at the beginning of colonial rule in 1844,[129] and the appointment of Ng as Legislative Councilor came only in 1880. The appointment of the first Chinese Executive Councilor Chow Shou Son was even later, not occurring until 1926.[130] It is worth noting, however, that the appointments in fact emerged out of the need for the colonial government to cope with the problem of illegitimacy. In turn, the elites were admitted into the political structure only as advisers to the government, rather than as decision makers.[131] The underlying political calculation was through the "administrative absorption of politics", King unravels how absorption went some way to legitimizing colonial rule,

> The government coopts the political forces, often represented by elite groups, into an administrative decision-making body, thus achieving some level of elite integration; as a consequence, the governing authority is made legitimate, and a loosely integrated political community is established.[132]

To ensure that the elites remain aligned with the goals of the government, only the emerging socioeconomic elites, who were "order-prosperity minded" and came from a narrow sector (business) of the Chinese population, were appointed.[133] The convergence of the government's and some elites' interests was achieved by the former carefully selecting elites who shared the same need to influence local society in terms of sanitation and urban order. Therefore, it is no surprise that the chosen elites represented their class interests more than those of the general Chinese public. To legitimize colonial rule, more JP and Legislative Councilor appointments followed: in 1882, three out of forty-nine nonofficial JPs were Chinese, including Ng Choy, Ho Kai and Wei Yuk, and more were appointed in the early twentieth century; by 1905, 17 out of 117 JPs were Chinese.[134] Meanwhile, Wong Shing, the founding director of TWH, became the second Chinese person to be appointed as a Legislative Councilor in the years 1884–90 and the second Chinese Sanitary Board member (1888–91).[135]

There were many more Chinese official appointments; Ng Choy's brother-in-law, Ho Kai, was the first Chinese Sanitary Board member (1886–1914) and the third Chinese Legislative Councilor to be appointed and is probably the most renowned Councilor (1890–1914) before the early twentieth century.[136] He began his career as a medical doctor and later as a barrister-in-law in the early 1880s, during which he developed his career in public service, starting with being a JP and then joining the Sanitary Board, Legislative Council and District Watch Committee.[137] Next, Wei Yuk, the son-in-law of Wong Shing, was the fourth person appointed as a Legislative Councilor (1896–1917). He was comprador to the Chartered Mercantile Bank of India, London and China, and he was knighted in 1919 as Sir Poshan Wei.[138] All four of these political appointees were educated in Britain, ensuring that they obtained some knowledge of Western practices and values while nonetheless maintaining the ability to look at colonial policies with Chinese eyes.[139] However, the number of appointees was small and the process was slow, sending the message that only a minority of Chinese, those who were successful in business or gained social influence, would be eligible for these crucial political resources.[140] Under this scarcity of such political capital, the government carefully allocated the resources in exchange for elites' cooperation in colonial governance.

Bearing all of this in mind while looking at Hennessy's pro-Chinese attitude, it is clear that he was certainly appreciated by Chinese elites. This explains why a year later, in 1881, a deputation of approximately 60 elites presented a congratulatory address in recognition of his fourth year governing the colony.[141] Many of this delegation were also compradors, landowners and top taxpayers, such as Kwok Acheong's son, Kwok Ying Kai (No. 8 taxpayer in 1881, contributing HK$5,748), Ip Ching Chuen (No. 17, HK$4,516, who was the comprador to the Hong Kong, Canton and Macao Steamboat Company), and Choy Chan (No. 18, HK$4,048).[142] Six were toilet landowners: Cheng Sing Yeung, Choy Chan, Ip Ching Chuen, Ng Sang, and Kwok Acheong's sons Kwok Yin Kai and Kwok Mui Kai represented him after his death in 1880. Prominent among these was Choy Chan, who owned 172 pieces of land in 1877, then 46 pieces in 1880, and his estate was worth one million Hong Kong dollars when registered in 1904.[143] Choy's great wealth was largely accumulated through investing in the highly profitable reclamation schemes of 1890 to 1904 in Central and Western districts, initiated by C. P. Chater, a notable Parsee real estate entrepreneur and Legislative Councilor.[144] With the opening of the Suez Canal in 1869, these two districts became very prosperous as the land became much more valuable for shipping, a process that was magnified by Hong Kong's naturally deep harbor.

Indeed, political appointments were a recognition of the prominent position of Chinese, as there was a firm belief that previous and continuing economic and political stability was largely based upon the investment and support of Chinese elites.[145] Being a partner in colonial governance was closely relevant to the Chinese population's growing recognition in the political sphere and was certainly a reflection of their growing economic capital. That is, when Chinese became economically powerful, it inevitably led to a higher degree of reliance on them by the government to sustain colonial rule, therefore building their political power. Obviously, the associated rise of wealth, elite status and political authority was not coincidental; rather, they were mutually reinforcing. Wealth may be used to obtain higher social status, and higher status helps acquire more resources, meaning wealth, which altogether usually has beneficial political consequences. More importantly, the Chinese were not purely objects and could make use of their economic and social capital to act as active agents to exert great leverage on the government and become involved in colonial governance.

2.5 Concluding Remarks

In a changing political-economic context, the new circumstances allowed new multi-layered interactions between the newly risen Chinese business elites and the government. Economic restructuring gave Chinese people opportunities to expand their wealth and land holdings. It was obvious that the Chinese were by no means holding still, the more adaptable ones were well positioned for the new chances arising from colonialism, successfully seizing the opportunities of the new political-economic context. Some of them were able to translate their economic and social capital into political capital and thus restructure their relationship with the government into one of collaborations, therefore capturing public power that was available due to the limitations of colonial rule. The taking up of a governance role by the Chinese elites was closely tied to the growing recognition of their economic and social capital, which was gained through the land market and trade, and the social influence cultivated from catering public services for the Chinese community.

The government and elites were both obliged to cooperate in colonial governance, as they had a shared self-interest in terms of economic development and social stability. Rear is correct to note that colonial collaboration in fact drew upon "strong common self-interest in public order and the economic stability which goes with it".[146] This was a pragmatic consideration of mutual self-interest, of which the function and sustainability of colonial rule rested. The elites benefitted from the collaboration in that it strengthened their political position by increasing their ability to intervene in colonial governance and reshape policies to their advantage. Based on self-interest, the relationship can be better understood as a resource interdependent relationship. This suggests that the government and elites could negotiate and maintain their relationship only as long as they were interdependent, that is, as long as they needed the resources of the other party to further their goals.

The extension of elites' influence from business-related areas into public services indicates the blurring of the traditional boundaries of colonizer-colonized and government-business. This reflects that the government was not necessarily fulfilling all public roles and that the elites could provide public services to become partners in public governance. In making such moves, the leading Chinese altered their role from being passive recipients, servants and subordinates into active, resourceful elites and governance partners, who formed not only an economic pillar of the colony but also came to be a political pillar. The collaborative role played by elites in providing such services was crucial to the sustainability of colonial rule and reflects the complexity of colonial relationships. Participation in public services helped to redefine their changing public role and interdependent relations with the government, which certainly made their involvement in colonial governance more dynamic and challenged the ideal colonial spatial order while engaging their land interests (rental and property exchange value) in public health, which we will see in the following chapters.

Notes

1. Chan, 1991; Chan, 1991; Law, 2009; Sinn, 2013; Tsai, 1993.
2. The declaration from Norton-Kyshe, 1971, Vol. 1. Financial arrangement from Endacott, 1964; Munn, 2009.
3. Revenue, CO129/6, 1844, p. 302–5. See also Endacott, 1964; Munn, 2009.
4. Bristow, 1984; Endacott, 1964; Lethbridge, 1978.
5. Opium revenue from revenue & resources of the colony, 29 June 1844, CO129/6, p. 303; Munn, 2009: 372. Land revenue from endnote 4.
6. Hong Kong Government, 1887: x.
7. Endacott, 1964: 54, 100.
8. Abstract of the Net Revenue and Expenditure of Hong Kong, *BB*, 1871–1877.
9. Abstract of the Net Revenue and Expenditure of Hong Kong, *BB*, 1878; Revenue and Expenditure, *BB*, 1879–1910.
10. Carroll, 2007: 49–52; Endacott, 1964: 116–7.
11. Carroll, 2007: 35.
12. Census, *GG*, 11 March 1853; Endacott, 1964: 116.
13. Population, *BB*, 1871, 1881, 1891.
14. Endacott, 1964: 65; Population, *BB*, 1891.
15. Chan, 1991; Evans, 1970.
16. Reports of the Medical Officer of Health, the Sanitary Surveyor, and the Colonial Veterinary Surgeon for the Year 1897, p. 270.
17. Chadwick, 1882.
18. Report on the Town of Victoria, Colonial Surgeon to Colonial Secretary, 15 April 1874. *Annual Report of the Colonial Surgeon for 1879*, No. 37, 1880.
19. Revenue, Governor Sir H. Robinson to Sir F. Rogers, Bart, May 21 1863. Enclosure 3 in No. 3, *BPP 1863–1881*, Vol. 25, 1971, p. 7.
20. AJPH, *GG*, 11 February 1882, p. 82.
21. Evans, 1970: 70; Munn, 2009: 95.
22. RCHK, Surveyor General to Colonial Secretary, 8 May 1877. Enclosure 1, in No.1; and Governor Hennessy to the Earl of Carnarvon, 27 September 1877. No. 1, *BPP 1863–1881*, Vol. 25, 1971, p. 647–50.
23. RCHK, Surveyor General to Colonial Secretary, 8 May 1877. Enclosure 1, in No.1; Minute by the Registrar General, 16 May 1877. Enclosure 3, in No.1, *BPP 1863–1881*, *BPP 1863–1881*, Vol. 25, 1971, p. 649, 651.
24. RCHK, Surveyor General to Colonial Secretary, 8 May 1877. Enclosure 1, in No.1; and Governor Hennessy to the Earl of Carnarvon, 27 September 1877. No. 1, *BPP 1863–1881*, Vol. 25, 1971, p. 647–50.
25. RCHK, Governor to the Earl, 27 September 1877. Enclosure 1, *BPP 1863–1881*, Vol. 25, 1971, p. 647–8.
26. For overcrowding, see Report on the Town of Victoria, Colonial Surgeon to Colonial Secretary, 15 April 1874. *Annual Report of the Colonial Surgeon for 1879*, No. 37, 1880; RCHK, Surveyor General to Colonial Secretary, 8 May 1877. Enclosure 1 in No.9, *BPP 1863–1881*, *BPP 1863–1881*, Vol. 25, 1971, p. 658–9. For open defecation, see RCHK, Governor Hennessy to the Earl of

Kimberley, 8 July1880. No.19, *BPP 1863–1881*, *BPP 1863–1881*, Vol. 25, 1971, p. 663.

27. Eitel, 1895; Endacott, 1964.
28. RCHK, Governor Hennessy to the Earl of Carnarvon, 8 July1880. No.19, *BPP 1863–1881*, *BPP 1863–1881*, Vol. 25, 1971, p. 663.
29. Munn, 2009; Pomfret, 2013.
30. Statement of Governor on the Census Returns, 3 June 1881. Enclosure 2 in No. 42, *BPP 1863–1881*, Vol. 25, 1971, p. 723.
31. Endacott, 1964; Lethbridge, 1978.
32. AJPH, GG, 11 February 1882, p. 82.
33. AJPH, *GG*, 11 February 1882, p. 80.
34. Carroll, 2007; Endacott, 1964; Smith, 1985.
35. Esherick and Rankin, 1990; Tsai, 1993.
36. Parkin, 1972.
37. Smith, 1971: 77.
38. Sinn, 2003; Tsai, 1993.
39. Smith, 1985.
40. Carroll, 2007; Hui, 1997; Tsai, 1993.
41. Statement of Governor on the Census Returns, 3 June 1881. Enclosure 2 in No. 42, *BPP 1863–1881*, Vol. 25, 1971, p. 724–5. See also Chan, 1991: 67.
42. Hui, 1997.
43. Statement of Governor on the Census Returns, 3 June 1881. Enclosure 2 in No. 42, *BPP 1863–1881*, 1971, Vol. 25, p. 731.
44. Chan, 1991; Endacott, 1964; Sinn, 2003.
45. Robinson, 1972: 142.
46. Eitel, 1895; Tsai, 1993.
47. Lau, 1982.
48. Lau, 1982.
49. Lau, 1982: 19.
50. Sinn, 2003: 4.
51. Munn, 2009; Rogaski, 2004; Yu, 2010; Trocki, 2006.
52. Munn, 2009: 99.
53. Munn, 2009: 99. More about the system from Davis to Stanley, 29 June 1844, CO129/6, p. 302–5.
54. Carroll, 2007; Munn, 2009.
55. Revenue & resources of the colony, 29 June 1844, CO129/6, p. 303.
56. The partnership from CS/I007/00064053.GIF, CS/I007/00064049.GIF, Carl Smith Collection. More about Li Sing and Li Tak Cheong from Carroll, 2007; Munn, 2009; Tsai, 1993.
57. Carroll, 2007: 51–3.
58. AJPH, *GG*, 11 February 1882, p. 82.
59. Carroll, 2007: 52.
60. No. 25, Li Tak-Cheong, *GG*, 15 February 1873.
61. *HKDP*, 24 February 1880; CS/I001/00006809.GIF, CS/I003/00029951.GIF, Carl Smith Collection.

62. Pennel, 1961.
63. List of directors from https://www.tungwah.org.hk/en/about/corporate-governance/board-of-directors/former-board-of-directors/.
64. CS/I003/00029959.GIF, Carl Smith Collection.
65. Carroll, 2007; Chan, 1991; Chu, 2013b; Sinn, 2003; Smith, 1971; Tsai, 1993.
66. Smith, 1985: 115.
67. Tang, 1996. This author, Tang Kwong Yan, is Tang Luk's great grandson.
68. Lo, 1971.
69. For his land holdings, the author calculated from those registered in the Hong Kong Rate Book, see HKRS38-2–33, *RB*, 1880. For the tax, see AJPH, *GG*, 11 February 1882, p. 82.
70. Probate, *BB*, 1888. For the tax, see AJPH, *GG*, 11 February 1882, p. 82.
71. Carroll, 2007; Chan, 1991; Sinn, 2003.
72. Tsai, 1993; Sinn, 2003.
73. Carroll, 2007; Lethbridge, 1978; Sinn, 2003; Tsai, 1993.
74. Midgal, 1988.
75. Chu, 2013b; Law, 2009; Sinn, 2003; Tsai, 1993.
76. Carroll, 2007; Chan, 1991; Munn, 2009.
77. Lethbridge, 1978: 113.
78. Carroll, 2007: 64.
79. Carroll, 2007: 64; Munn, 2009: 369; Tsai, 1993: 61.
80. Munn, 2009; Carroll, 2007.
81. Lethbridge, 1978: 58.
82. No. 199, Victoria Registration, *GG*, 12 December 1874.
83. Chadwick, 1882; Carroll, 2007.
84. Carroll, 2007: 65; Lethbridge, 1978: 109.
85. Carroll, 2007; Tsai, 1993.
86. Mills, 1942: 398.
87. Carroll, 2007: 137.
88. Chan, 1991; Munn, 2009; Sinn, 2003; Tsai, 1993.
89. Acting Colonial Secretary to Messrs. Lo, Lai-ping, *GG*, 3 July 1880, No. 723, p. 518. More about PLK from Carroll, 2007; Lethbridge, 1978; Munn, 2009.
90. Carroll, 2007: 63; Sinn, 2003: 133–6.
91. Chan, 1991; Tsai, 1993; but Sinn suggests another argument that the elites were in fact compelled to collaborate with the government, see Sinn, 2013.
92. Carroll, 2007; Sinn, 2003.
93. Tsai, 1993: 69.
94. Carroll, 2007; Chan, 1991; Law, 2009; Sinn, 2003; Tsai, 1993.
95. Sinn, 2003.
96. Tung Wah Hospital, *GG*, 16 February 1878, p. 47.
97. Sinn, 2003.
98. Tobin, 1999: 22.
99. Law, 2009; Sinn, 2003.
100. Carroll, 2007: 34.
101. Eitel, 1895.

102. Carroll, 2007: 22.
103. Carroll, 2007; Munn, 2009.
104. *HKDP*, 21 October 1865, 18 January 1869.
105. Olympia, *HKDP*, 1 October 1878. See also Carroll, 2007; Coates, 1980.
106. Holdsworth and Munn, 2012; The Surveyor General to Kwok Acheong, HKRS 419–2-203, 1859.
107. Tung Wah Hospital, *GG*, 16 February 1878.
108. Chinese Deputation to the Governor, *GG*, 24 February, 1880; Enclosure 2 in No. 42, *BPP*, Vol. 25, p. 724.
109. *HKDP*, 12 May 1880.
110. Carroll, 2007: 18.
111. Law, 2009: 15.
112. AJPH, *GG*, 11 February 1882, p. 82.
113. CS/I004/00035685.GIF; CS/I004/00036653.GIF, Carl Smith Collection.
114. CS/I004/00036697.GIF, Carl Smith Collection.
115. Smith, 1971: 100. See also CS/I004/00036655.GIF, Carl Smith Collection.
116. Chinese Houses, *GG*, 27 July 1878, p. 370–2.
117. Chinese Houses, *GG*, 27 July 1878, p. 372.
118. Ip Chuk-kai, HKRS 144–4-2183, 1901.
119. CS/I003/00026199.GIF, Carl Smith Collection.
120. List of directors from https://www.tungwah.org.hk/en/about/corporate-governance/board-of-directors/former-board-of-directors/. List of taxpayer from AJPH, *GG*, 11 February 1882, p. 82. Compradors from Smith, 1971 and 1985.
121. TWH, 1970: 163.
122. Chan, 1991; Sinn, 2003.
123. Statement of Governor on the Census Returns, 1881. Enclosure 2 in No. 42, China. *BPP 1863–1881*, Vol. 25, p. 728.
124. JP from The Justices of the Peace, *GG*, 24 December 1878, p. 599. Councilor from Ng Choy, *GG*, 2 June 1880, No. 130.
125. His background from Endacott, 1964. His speech from Tung Wah Hospital, *GG*, 16 February 1878.
126. CS/I003/00026196.GIF, Carl Smith Collection.
127. Endacott, 1973.
128. Sinn, 2003: 88.
129. Endacott, 1964: 43.
130. King, 1975: 426.
131. Tsai, 1993.
132. King, 1975: 424.
133. Chan, 1991; Sinn, 2003; Tsai, 1993.
134. The Justices of the Peace, *GG*, 21 January 1882, p. 20; The Justices of the Peace, *GG*, 3 March 1905, p. 186.
135. Endacott, 1964.
136. Choa, 1981; Lethbridge, 1978.
137. Carroll, 2007; Lethbridge, 1978.
138. Lethbridge, 1978.

139. Endacott, 1964; Lethbridge, 1978.
140. Chan 1991.
141. Congratulatory Address, *GG*, 23 April 1881, p. 274–6.
142. Tax from AJPH, *GG*, 11 February 1882, p. 82. Ip from HKRS144-4–764.
143. For land holdings, the author calculated from those registered in the Hong Kong Rate Book, see HKRS38-2–23, *RB*, 1877; HKRS38-2–33, *RB*, 1880. Choy's estate from Choy Chan, HKRS 144–4-1772, 1905; Probate, *BB*, 1905.
144. Choy's participation in the reclamation from Choy Chan, HKRS 144–4-1772, 1905. More about the project from Endacott, 1964; Bristow, 1984.
145. Lau, 1982; Tsai, 1991.
146. Rear, 1971: 78–9.

Chapter 3 Governing Urban Space: Racial and Class Politics

> Fortunately, in England, there is a public opinion against which even the rights of property, when wrongfully exercised, have to give way; at Hong Kong, property is the main consideration amongst a community that only congregates here to accumulate sufficient means…the so-called vested rights of property should very heavily handicap any effort of government at sanitation.[1]
>
> Acting Governor, Major General W. G. Cameron

3.1 Overview

Cameron made this comment during the tug of war between the government, Chinese landowners and politicians over the *Public Health Bill* in 1887. One aim of the *Bill* was the mandatory inclusion of domestic toilets in newly constructed dwellings.[2] He argued that the issue was that landowners, obsessed with land value, were resistant to health-related regulations rather than the government being reluctant to improve hygiene. However, it is somewhat simplistic to blame landowners, who were entangled in interests of value, to hamper the provision. Nevertheless, Cameron pinpointed the contradiction between regulation and profit accumulation that was operating on urban space in Hong Kong at the time, a contradiction embedded in land-centered capitalism. Complicating this further are the multiple internal class divisions within the Chinese and European public bodies and within the government over sanitation, interplaying racial and class politics. This chapter argues that a new conception of urban hygiene linked to economics emerged, which led to the reconfiguration of moral geography and set the stage for a capitalist turn of sanitation. By connecting the complexity of colonial relations to the inherent contradictions between spatial regulation and profit accumulation of urban space, it explores racial and class politics in governing colonial space. Much is at stake; the analysis sheds light on the entanglement of capitalism, morality and space over sanitation, which was influential in the blending of economic and moral logics.

To investigate the politics, it is first necessary to obtain an idea of the urban hygiene discourse. To show this, this chapter briefly examines how lower-class Chinese and

Y. Chong, *Toilet as Business for the Hygiene of the Chinese Community in Colonial Hong Kong*, https://doi.org/10.1007/978-981-19-1396-9_3

the Chinese quarter were cast as unhygienic, and sanitation infrastructure was configured as a morally charged space to regulate these Chinese people's use of space. After that, the chapter teases out the complex forces of capitalism, colonialism and ethnicity that influenced the urban hygiene discourse and the ideal colonial spatial order. To this end, the author first outlines the spatial connection of the Chinese quarter with disease within a colonial governmentality framework. This shows how the fear of disease bore negative associations with Chinese spaces and discusses the logic of colonial urbanism and the ethical role that was projected onto public toilets as a spatial technology to address sanitary problems and exercise morel governance on Chinese. Second, the author unravels the complex spatial relation between the government and Chinese beyond colonial governmentality by illustrating the characteristics of the capitalist form of sanitation in the colonies that was initiated jointly by them. This relationship made sanitation infrastructure not only a moral space but also a means of production.

3.2 Construction of Urban Hygiene Moral Discourse

It must be noted that political factors interacted to construct the colonial urban hygiene moral discourse in terms of connecting complex racial relationships: the lifestyle and hygiene practices of the Chinese community were politically well connected with disease by the government. Through a narrative study of such a connection, moral discourse can be better understood in light of racial politics.

3.2.1 The Health Connection Between Chinese, Disease and Urban Space

Soon after the establishment of the colony, there were frequent epidemics in Hong Kong. However, there is probably one key occasion that brought the colonial government's attention to the local sanitary condition; this was the outbreak of "Hong Kong Fever" in the summer of 1843, soon after the colony was established.[3] European civilians and garrisons were both severely affected by the outbreak, with 10% of civilians and 24% of troops dying between May and October 1843.[4] However, utmost attention was directed to the high death rate within the garrison. A total of 60 troops died in ten weeks at the West Point Barracks (above Pokfulam Road, which was close to Chinese areas),[5] and throughout 1843, one-third (440 troops) died of disease, as mentioned in Chap. 1. The cause of the disease was identified to be miasma from decaying animals and vegetation matter, which was disposed of by Chinese individuals in areas surrounding their neighborhood. The underlying problem was that Chinese people tended to neglect hygiene, which stemmed from their dirty habits and inferior morals.[6] Chinese people and their spaces were seen by the government as the origin of the disease outbreaks, so the people who lived there were treated as dangerous and a threat to urban order.[7]

Within a spatial imaginary of sanitation, the worsening health of Europeans and garrisons was linked with the appalling conditions of the Chinese community. Here, the government identified the locus of the disease to be the Chinese public and their spaces, which was then translated into a guideline for the location of barracks in the city. As Cowell notes, "a mantle of doubt and fear seemed to extend itself upon the very terrain of the land itself…becoming an almost precise set of rules about where to build and how to build".[8] This certainly alerted the military to the sanitary condition of the Chinese community, who lived close to barracks. In the midst of the outbreak, the Major General, A. F. Saltoun, made a complaint to Governor H. Pottinger (1841–44), noting the health risk of a village community toilet being near the Stanley Barracks. Pottinger soon prohibited any such facility in the vicinity of any barracks.[9]

The confluence of an epidemic and the nuisances of miasma was perceived as a specific urban crisis, which aroused much concern from the government and British press.[10] It is not surprising that the press campaigned for a better environment; seeking methods to manage the Chinese public and their spaces was a popular subject in newspapers.[11] The great anxiety about the dangers of being proximate to the Chinese entailed a critical relation between Chinese, disease and urban space, after which a particular moral discourse of urban hygiene was formulated to govern the urban landscape. Colonial urbanism as a means of social control and segregation was very proficient at "Othering" along lines of race and establishing boundaries that segregated locals and their space while identifying such spaces to be immoral and unhygienic.[12] The Hong Kong colonial government followed suit; it deployed the combined spatial technologies of segregation, with a focus on controlling Chinese bodies' relationship to urban space and moral geography, with a focus on inducing moral sanitary habits amongst Chinese.

Amongst the fear of another disease outbreak and many more deaths, the government used urban renewal projects to segregate Chinese people from Europeans and military infrastructure from urban areas. One such project, which turned the Upper Bazaar (an area opposite today's Central Market in Central District) into a business district, started in 1844 and lasted to the early 1850s.[13] Indeed, the Bazaar located at the heart of the city generated considerable land revenue for the government. However, its concern went far beyond revenue, and the project also responded to concerns over sanitation and urban order that were expressed in a particular view of the regulation of urban space. Sanitation and order were seen in light of the racial and class differences of the colonial context. The government portrayed this class of Chinese as an intrusive group who invaded a district once occupied by respectable Chinese and as people who were engaged in immoral activities, such as gambling. Their behavior was considered to be a nuisance in the neighborhood, opposing the perceived colonial urban order of neatness and safety.[14] Concerns about disorder fostered political demands for urban regulation, and it was argued that these Chinese were a menace to order. A committee consisting of the Chief Magistrate, Chinese Secretary and Land Officer was formed, and they were entrusted with the task of moving the Chinese out of the city center westward to the Taipingshan area (around modern day Hollywood Road and Taipingshan Street) where a considerable number of Chinese had already settled; this area gradually became the colony's Chinatown.[15]

The government claimed that the Upper Bazaar project was a renewal project that sought to increase land revenue and ensure the proper use of urban space, but the attitudes and actions present were obviously racial. Chinese, regardless of class, were not permitted to occupy houses in the new district. This binary spatial arrangement marginalized Chinese at the lower-western part of the city, as such it was manifested in an obsession with boundaries and segregation. The essential point is that altitude and location were prime concerns of the government. The Upper Bazaar, also known as "Mid-levels" and situated above Central District, was at an altitude that allowed fresh air to circulate freely through the streets. Fresh air was believed to drive away miasma, and the area was regarded as desirable and healthy. At the time, there was a tendency among colonial governments to perceive height as a guarantee of sanitary conditions in tropical colonies.[16] It should be no surprise that as in the other colonial societies,[17] the Chinese were not passive objects that could be easily manipulated to conform to colonial spatial ordering. In practice, they were resentful of their discriminatory removal and restriction and petitioned for the government to compensate for their loss.[18] Nonetheless, the issue was resolved with compensation, but the high concentration of Chinese in a certain area actually came to undermine the colony's overall sanitation. For the government, however, indecent living styles (e.g., overcrowding) and bodily behavior (e.g., public defecation) were two factors largely responsible for turning the Chinese quarter into a disease breeding ground. The government's views, however, were laid in a belief of Chinese people's inability to self-consciously control their bodies, meaning that Chinese people lacked concern for urban hygiene.

3.2.2 Indecent Living Styles

Beginning in the early 1850s, population growth was particularly high, as the rapid urbanization of the colony, development of international trade and broadening of the entrepot base meant that there were more opportunities incoming migrants.[19] Seeing the benefit of colonial rule and the disturbance caused by the Taiping Rebellion during the early 1850s and mid-1860s, both poor and wealthy mainland Chinese flocked to Hong Kong to earn a living or try their luck at acquiring a fortune.[20] The population significantly increased from a few thousand to 39,000 between 1841 and 1853. Since then, the population has grown by 25 to 34% each decade in the second half of the nineteenth century.[21] By the late nineteenth century, approximately 160,000 Chinese resided in Victoria City, two-thirds of which were settled in the lower-western part of the city, as shown in Chap. 2. With the outbreak of the 1911 revolution in China, the influx of Chinese people further pushed the population up to 456,739.[22] Population growth in the early twentieth century accelerated further, with an average annual increase of 15,000 people from 1901 to 1921.[23]

Rapid population growth in a small area highly distorted the supply and demand of housing, which resulted in housing shortages and price hikes. Such a situation garnered the interest of both European and Chinese property speculators and enabled them to build low-cost and poorly designed tenement houses.[24] As land was so expensive, land developers modified the typical housing design of Chinese and British single- or multistory houses to minimize the loss of rental space and accommodate more tenants. Three main modifications to a typical urban house were employed.[25] First, houses were constructed in blocks, back to back without yards, with narrow street frontages, and they only had windows on the street side. Due to the low building cost, this type of house had been widely built in Britain since the early nineteenth century.[26] Second, houses had narrow gullies at the back. Third, the backs of cellular floors were formed of the ground of the street above, owing to the steep nature of the ground on which the houses were built. The average size of such a tenement was 26 by 14 feet, with 10 foot ceilings, this was partitioned into eight cubicle homes which averaged 7 by 6 feet in area, and 7 feet high, the remaining 3 feet of height being converted into a loft.[27] However, being cheap to build did not mean they were cheap to rent. In the 1870s, a house in Hong Kong with three rooms each approximately 14 square feet, with a poor kitchen, would rest for between £55 and £70 per year. The rent in Hong Kong was even higher than that in London.[28] On average, each tenement contained five to ten families, each paying a monthly rent ranging from £2.1 to £5.[29] High pressure on rent and their design intensified overcrowding. This resulted in population densities of 400–1,000 persons per acre being reached in some areas of the Chinese quarter by 1897.[30]

Clearly, the immediate solution to the housing shortage, building cheap and intensive accommodations, was rooted in harmful profiteering. As a result, these buildings undoubtedly contributed to the ill effects of overcrowding, undermining general cleanliness.[31] It is well known that cramped living conditions exacerbate poor hygiene in the course of daily living; for example, the compressed house designs made it difficult for air to circulate, and even worse was the smoke from cooking pervading the houses. Such living conditions predispose inhabitants to disease; if a number of sick people are crowded together in close, dirty, and unventilated houses, the disease will spread easily. Much evidence shows a correlation between the increase in mortality and the increase in the density of back-to-back houses in early twentieth-century Britain.[32] This not only encouraged disease but also overcrowding caused general physical and mental harm, as living conditions made it difficult to care for oneself or live with dignity.

However, the causes of overcrowding in the Chinese quarter were complex, and the disease was seen to be caused by Chinese habits rather than by poor housing conditions due to property speculation and spatial segregation. The view of overcrowding involved an emphasis on Chinese moral deficiency of singling out their living style. The government considered overcrowding to be a part of Chinese people's chosen culture: "breathing seems to be optional…We hear much of Chinese overcrowding, but overcrowding is the normal condition of the Chinese, and they do not appear to be inconvenienced by it at all".[33] Again, men, women and children lived together with dogs and pigs in damp, dark and unventilated rooms, which was seen by British as a dangerous kind of irrationality. The Chinese rationality was that they could feed the pigs their food scraps and then sell the pig and earn much-needed income. The Chinese probably knew it was less than ideal for keeping animals like farms in such cramp conditions; however, they had no choice because they were so poor. In a sense, it was a rational thing to keep pigs in their living situation which created this circumstance to store value, but such practices were unacceptable from the colonial governing perspective and assumed the Chinese were just inferior, even though similar practices were found amongst the lower-class in nineteenth-century Britain.[34] In 1880, the Colonial Surgeon, P. B. Ayres, stated his surprise that 172 pigs were kept under the beds of one tenement building, and his comment was it "would not be considered fit to put pigs in by any decent person".[35] The living style of lower-class Chinese further focused the government's attention on their bodily behaviour, and the lack of domestic toilets was one of the first problems to be confronted.

3.2.3 Public Defecation

The density of dwellings and people made the demand for toilets acute, while poor-quality tenement houses generally lacked domestic toilets.[36] In lieu of toilets, alternative solutions such as night soil buckets were commonly used. In most cases, buckets kept under the bed were emptied every two to three days; hence, miasma was certainly seen to be a significant risk.[37] Furthermore, was the constructions of improvised toilets in kitchens, which reflects Chinese were well aware of the needs to address the daily necessities in the urban city. However, it must be noted that even people with good sanitary behavior could not properly exercise in a seriously poor situation. Colonial Surgeon, Ayres was in despair over the sanitation in one tenement building after an inspection in 1874. He wrote,

> In the kitchens were generally one or more hutches used as privies, consisting of a few boards knocked together to form a rickety screen, and from age and neglect they were saturated with filth. No proper receptacle for night-soil was found in these hutches, - sometimes a broken pot, sometimes a leaky old tub, sometimes nothing at all, the night soil being deposited on the floor and the urine draining away, as best it might, into the surrounding floors. I've a pretty good stomach and don't stick at trifles, but I found the inspection of these places acted as a very unpleasant emetic.[38]

Seeing the poor sanitary conditions of the houses and witnessing three disease outbreaks in a week in April 1874, Ayres left a note of caution that outbreaks would become more frequent in the Chinese quarter.[39] Despite the potential health risks of living in these substandard houses, they satisfied both property speculators and tenants. Speculators were pleased by the low construction costs, while this did not mean cheap rentals, as shown in the previous chapter. The tenants, mainly coolies, were satisfied with the availability of the housing. However, without proper hygiene facilities in the buildings, the most commonly sought alternative was gutters and back lanes, and so many public areas in the Chinese quarter were generally in dirty condition.[40] The Colonial Surgeon, J. C. Dempster, first warned the ill effect of public defecation and insanitary conditions in Taipingshan, a district in the quarter. He wrote in his annual report dated 1854 that,

> [Taipingshan was in] A most objectionable state, containing almost invariably cowsheds, pigsties, stagnant pools - the receptacles of every kind of filth, all which nuisances have remained unheeded for a considerable time...great complaints are made of the offensive effluvia (dripping through the walls) by almost every European passer-by...Nothing can be more offensive than the laying out to dry of large quantities of manure on small patches of ground in the rear of this locality...the emanations from which not only interfere with the pleasantness of a walk much frequented by the inhabitants of Hongkong, but must be sources of annoyance to those living in the adjacent neighborhood.[41]

The underlying message was that miasma emanating from bodily waste was injurious not only to Chinese peoples' health but also to the neighborhoods' and the colony as a whole. This underlined the colonial perception of the dangers of living close to lower-class Chinese and the slum-Chinese quarter. It was accepted among the government that there was a chain of disease transmission that began at Chinese people living in the quarter and then went to Indian troops, European seamen and garrison troops, prisoners, and finally upper class Europeans.[42] In the dimension of colonial governance, public defecation was reflected in class and race as a deficiency of the lower-class Chinese body and mind, who were unable to control their bodily functions.

The dirt out of place that the Chinese produced was then conceived beyond the actual diseases that they caused and instead conceived in terms of the threat of disorder itself. Therefore, the inability to defecate in the correct place was not seen as an affliction of poverty or living conditions but rather as a sign of immoral noncompliance with the correct ordering of body and space. Bodily waste was no longer seen as a natural product of a human being; rather, it was depicted as hostile to the body and space. As noted earlier from Douglas, dirt is "matter out of place" and so becomes explicitly moral. Following this logic, improper Chinese sanitary habits and living styles were seen as part of a wider syndrome of antisocial behavior and were an issue of immorality. Therefore, their bodily waste left in public areas was regarded as both physical and moral pollution. From this view, the government was very concerned about the ways in which Chinese used open space under pragmatic and moral terms. The demand for toilets became an urgent issue to address the daily necessities of poor Chinese. In 1854, the Colonial Surgeon, Dempster, urged "a great want of Privies and suitable Depots for dirt is observable everywhere the Native population reside", that the demand was first impressed upon the government.[43]

Many sanitarians had a keen concern for the problem of public defecation. The reality that much was at stake is reflected in the complaint from Colonial Surgeon, Ayres, who was worried about defecation near government house and the racket court in the center of Victoria City.[44] Threats to public health continued to strengthen the stereotype that lower-class Chinese were producers of disease and their spaces were disease-ridden, which reconfirmed racial and class prejudices while heightening the sense that these Chinese were a race apart and detrimental to general health in the colony. Nevertheless, the real causes behind the outbreaks were complex. The spread of disease was accelerated by the lack of proper hygiene facilities and cramp housing conditions, which was an issue not just in the Chinese quarter; it was bad everywhere, which helped it spread. However, the particularly poor living conditions amongst Chinese spurred further spatial segregation between Chinese and Europeans. The wave of opposition from government officials and the War Office against Governor Hennessy allowing Chinese people to purchase houses in European areas between 1877 and 1880 was obviously linked to this stereotype.

In 1877, the Registrar General and the Protector of the Chinese, S. C. Smith, argued that the differing structures of Chinese and European houses were essentially due to the respective customs, habits, and living style of each ethnicity.[45] What worried him was that the rental yield of European houses (compared to Chinese houses) would be lower among Chinese houses than among European houses. More opposition from the War Office, the most significant of which probably comes from Major General, E. W. Donovan, who often clashed with Hennessy, strongly objected to small Chinese lodgings being in the vicinity of any barracks on sanitary grounds.[46] The first reason for Donovan's opposition was dense living conditions. If there were any outbreaks of disease, it would spread much faster if people were living closer together. Any rapid spread would be disastrous to the nearby garrison. The second concern was about insanitary Chinese behaviors, which included making use of open space behind houses as a toilet. As a result of his concerns, Donovan urged the resumption of 95 houses (occupied by 3,000 Chinese) between the Murray and Victoria Barracks, located in Central China. This suggestion would have cost HK$20,000, one-tenth fall government annual revenue, and hence was ignored by government.[47] In return, Hennessy criticized that the Major General was prejudiced against Chinese; nonetheless, a large number of dilapidated Chinese houses were replaced with "superior, first class Chinese dwellings".[48] Despite Hennessy winning this battle by allowing Chinese to purchase houses in the European area, as noted in the previous chapter, the War Office definitely did not accept his argument, leading to two consequences.

The first came from Lord Kimberley, the newly appointed Principal Secretary of State for the Colonies, who appointed Obsert Chadwick to carry out an investigation into the sanitary conditions in Hong Kong in 1881.[49] One focus of his investigation was that the provision of public toilets shall be explained more later. The second consequence was the enactment of the *European District Reservation Ordinance* in 1888, after Hennessy's term as governor had ended.[50] This ordinance restricted Chinese houses from being built above Caine Road, thus reserving the hill area on Hong Kong Island exclusively for Europeans. Clearly, segregation was achieved by the regulation of building types that were actually associated with sanitary habits along racial lines. The original housing rules approved by Hennessy only allowed Chinese people to purchase houses below Caine Road. While this was nonetheless an extension of the area that Chinese were allowed to purchase within, it nonetheless reinforced existing spatial segregation. The 1888 Ordinance moved a step further by explicitly prohibiting Chinese habitation above Caine Road, introducing a perception of a protective barrier for Europeans. The use of law is important because it affected what Swanson notes: "[that] sanitation syndrome was a force in its own right" and provided a legal means to exercise segregation and social control.[51] Following this, the *Ordinance for the Reservation of a Residential Area in the Hill District* was passed in 1904, which extended the prohibited hill areas.[52] These ordinances stressed the importance of altitude for the protection of Europeans' health and further relegated Chinese to the Chinese quarter. The result was an intensification of the problems resulting from overcrowding and poor sanitation in the Chinese area. The fear of disease and the health connection between Chinese and European continued to drive spatial segregation and close surveillance of Chinese bodies and their use of urban space. This raises the question of the means to monitor and guide Chinese in the proper use of space.

3.3 Moral Geography: Colonial Public Toilets

In parallel with the traditional spatial segregation of disorderly space, there was the introduction of new techniques and new sites of governance to regulate urban space. Through reorganizing internal space, which made lower-class Chinese easier to surveil, the colonial public toilets were staged moral spaces for manifesting colonial disciplinary measures and moral governance. This form of governing emphasized moral improvement of the body and space under the hope of inducing conscious and moral bodily control in terms of the "proper" use of space to achieve cleanliness. As Wohl says, "public health was always more than just a movement for social reform—it took on the intensity of a mission".[53] This mission was complicated in colonies because colonial rule regarded public health provisions as a moral force to cure pathological others. As McFarlane argues, sanitation infrastructure serves as a technology of rule as both a material and discursive object in colonies.[54] It was within the rubric of a moralizing mission that toilets were seen as an answer to racial and class deficiencies, bringing lower-class Chinese habits into conformity with European civilizing and progressive values under the government's guidance.

3.3.1 Managing Chinese Bodily Behaviors

Managing Chinese bodily habits such as public defecation through toilet provision was first impressed upon the government in 1854, but it did become urgent until the sudden outbreaks of ague, dysentery and fever between February and May 1856. Of the 799 Chinese deaths, 379 (48%) and 155 (19%) were living in Taipingshan and the Lower Bazaar (today Sheung Wan), two crowded districts in the Chinese quarter.[55] The adjacent Upper Bazaar, inhabited by Europeans, also registered 111 deaths (14%), causing great anxiety that Europeans would be widely exposed to disease. These events finally focused the government's attention on the "waste-disposal problem", and they urgently enacted the *Buildings and Nuisances Ordinance*, which provided a legal framework for the provision of public toilets (either a privy, urinal or water closet) to the Surveyor General.[56] However, no toilets were provided.

The *Buildings and Nuisances Ordinance* also included stipulations about toilet provision inside of dwellings. It required property developers to include domestic toilets in their new builds, and those in contravention of this *ordinance* were deemed a nuisance and could be fined HK$50 to $100. Clearly, the government hoped to shift municipal responsibility to developers, with the hope that the business sector would bear the burden and solve the problem. However, the situation developed in the opposite direction. There are several reasons behind this. First, the *ordinance* was entirely copied from Britain's 1844 *Metropolitan Building Act*; however, a system of privies and water closets was out of place in Hong Kong. Nonetheless, community pail toilets were found in some Chinese villages, as noted in Stanley, although they were not comprehensive. Second, the most likely toilet provision was a single toilet to be shared amongst all the tenants of a single tenement building. However, this conflicted with Chinese culture, where it was improper for women to share a toilet with other people (especially men) even coming from the same family. Third, the high land price policy adopted in the colony made toilet provision exceptionally expensive compared to other cities at the time. The well-known Chinese phrase "land has its value" can explain the difficulty; providing a toilet increased a building's construction cost.

To make matters worse, the effectiveness of the *ordinance* was undermined by opposition to the heavy noncompliance fines.[57] Opposition came to a head, and a Memorial was signed by 19 Chinese and 60 European landowners, who argued the *Ordinance* would make property investors lose confidence in their investments. The memorialists included Kwok Acheong, Wei Kwong, who was the father of Wei Yuk, and the taipans of Dents & Co and Jardine, Matheson & Co. In November, a protest strike by both Chinese and European merchants took place. The government saw the need to lessen the tension and avoid the protest turning into a political issue, so they therefore mostly appeased the petitioners. This political pressure slowed the provision of such domestic toilets; as shown earlier, domestic toilets were rare, and cookhouses were instead often used for a pail toilet arrangement.

Rapid and large-scale urban growth, however, quickly worsened the state of sanitation, and the rate of admission to the hospital among Chinese individuals was higher than that among Europeans in the 1860s (Table 3.1). More specifically, during the repeated outbreak of yellow fever in March 1865 and March 1866, the Victoria Goal registered an extraordinarily 777 cases and 63 deaths.[58] It was believed that Taipingshan, which was largely inhabited by the poorest Chinese, was the disease source, as most infected came from there, so the new outbreak between 1865–1866 also took a racial and class character. The most alarming was the rate of sickness and mortality among garrisons, which has remained significant since the early 1860s (Table 3.2). After the ordinance was relaxed, disease outbreaks continued in 1864 and 1865, there was dramatic growth in hospital admissions among garrisons; 3,409 and 4,698 cases were admitted to the hospital, and the sickness rate jumped from 173.2% to 293.7%, respectively.[59] This high rate above 100% meant that a single soldier was repeatedly devastated by disease each year; as a result, the death toll increased from 68 to 121, and the mortality rate for troops increased from 3.4 to 7.6 between 1864 and 1865.

Table 3.1 Rate of admission to hospital of European and Chinese, 1859–66

	Total admissions	Europeans admitted	Chinese admitted
1859	8.6	6.0	28.1
1860	6.9	9.3	8.3
1861	6.5	9.2	11.7
1862	5.4	5.4	12.8
1863	10.6	10.1	32.3
1864	9.6	11.0	22.8
1865	12.2	7.3	20.7
1866	12.2	6.7	33.6

Source CSR for 1859–66, *GG,* 17 March 1866, p. 125; 23 March 1867, p. 102

Table 3.2 Sickness and mortality of the troops

Year	Strength (person)	Admissions to hospital (person)	Sickness (%)	Death (person)	Mortality (%)
1863	1,495	2,751	184.0	51	3.4
1864	1,964	3,409	173.2	68	3.4
1865	1,600	4,698	293.7	121	7.6
1866	1,132	2,690	237.6	39	3.5
1867	1,120	1,700	151.8	37	3.3

Source CSR for 1863–1867, *GG,* 9 April 1864, p. 128; 1 April 1865, p. 160; 17 March 1866, p. 125; 23 March 1867, p. 99; 22 February 1868, p. 57

The sudden increased morality alarmed that the government, in mid-March 1866, Governor R. G. MacDonnell, urgently appointed a Special Commission on Sanitary Condition to investigate the defective drainage system and serious overcrowding. The Commission was significant and consisted of the Colonial Secretary, Colonial Surgeon, Major General commanding the Forces, Deputy Inspector General of Hospitals, Naval Commander-in-Chief.[60] In a submission, the Inspector of Nuisances expressed desperation to the Commission at the insanitary condition of Taipingshan, which he found difficult to end, because it was

> … a very dirty place; the drains leading from the houses to the main drains are occasionally out of repair but not generally. The dirty state of this district is due to rubbish of all kinds being thrown into the street. There are no water closets, the excrement is taken away in buckets from the houses, in some instances deposited in reservoirs; one large one is near the New Theatre. The order is that this deposit should take place before 8 A.M. but this is not strictly adhered to; does not consider the sanitary state of this district has been improved, owing to the dirty habits of the people, and the difficulty of obtaining Summonses, as also from the lenient nature of the sentences of the Magistrates. Has been found fault with by the Magistrates for bringing before them so many very poor people who could not afford to pay fines, this has occurred several times, men have been frequently discharged as the Magistrate considered them to be too poor to pay a fine and that it was duty with the assistance of the

convicts to keep the place clean. The Magistrate has repeated this several times and witness [the Inspector] finds that for these reasons he is unable to do his duty at all.[61]

Above all, the sanitary conditions were miserable. The inspector condemned lower-class Chinese as a hopelessly filthy race that did not uphold their social responsibility of either keeping living spaces clean or strictly abiding by the night soil removal schedule. For the inspector, the low morality of Chinese made the lack of a toilet system and the inefficacy of a traditional night soil disposal method more injurious in a densely populated place such as Taipingshan. Worse still, the trouble of obtaining summons and the lenience of the magistrates refusing to prosecute undermining the inspector's effort to maintain cleanliness. It is noteworthy that this condemnation highlighted the racial deficiency of Chinese by the inspector, which created a sense of urgent government great intervention in the daily life of the Chinese.

3.3.2 *The Introduction of Government Public Toilets*

Health ordinances were attempted by the government, but alone were ineffective at regulating poor Chinese behavior, such as the first health ordinance. The *Ordinance for the Preservation of Good Order and Cleanliness* was passed in 1844, which prohibited any person from laying any offensive matter (dirt, dung and rubbish) in public areas, and those who violated this were liable to a penalty not exceeding £5.[62] Furthermore, no later than the early 1860s, the government made it clear that no one could obey calls of nature near a public way or stream.[63] However, the problem of public waste remained. In the 1860s, approximately 4,000 to 5,000 notices issued for the accumulation of filth or obstructed/defective drainage, two main problems stemming from high urban density. Prosecution was pursued less frequently, and the summons finally issued were limited (Table 3.3). The inspector of nuisances' condemnation was useful for the government that he pointed to the difficulties in

Table 3.3 Notice and summon issued by the inspector of Nuisances, 1863–67

Year	Notice (no.)	Obstruction and defective drainage (no.)	Accumulation of filth (no.)	Summon (no.)	Fined (person)	Discharged (person)	Fines (HK$)
1863	5,510	1,939	3,533	1,324	1,523	114	1,335
1864	5,084	2,074	3,010	3,024	2,965	59	2,192
1865	5,300	1,965	3,335	1,486	1,153	328	1,174.8
1866	4,621	163	4,458	1,754	1,466	288	1,053.1
1867	4,413	216	4,197	1,068	1,029	39	2,471.8

Source CSR for1863-8, *GG*, 9 April 1864, p.126; 1 April 1865, p. 171; 17 March 1866, p. 133; 23 March 1867, p. 107; 22 February 1868, p. 64

carrying out his duty, which justified with the strongest necessity, close surveillance of lower-class Chinese. The report was published in May 1866, and the chairman of the Commission, W. Dick, concluded that "the sanitary condition of Taipingshan is such as to require, the most active supervision".[64]

By 1866, the number of hospital admissions and deaths caused by disease among the garrisons had largely decreased; however, the sickness rate remained high at over 200% (Table 3.1). As noted, the health of the military was of utmost concern to the British government, so the continuing excessive sickness rate alarmed the British Parliament, which responded with an enquiry led by the House of Commons.[65] The issue was significant enough to add pressure to the idea of establishing government toilets. Finally, in 1867, the Hong Kong colonial government put the public toilet on the agenda, which emerged as a part of a wider planned sanitary regime that aimed to regulate Chinese bodily behaviours.[66] At this point, it is useful to note that public health initiatives not only need to be rationalized by a health crisis or social changes but also may be driven by the government's interests.[67] There is some truth that the demand for toilets was pressing, as rapid urbanization intensified the pressure from a growing population, causing dire sanitation risks as disease repeatedly devastated the Chinese quarter, significantly raising death rates among the lower class. However, a combination of political factors interacted to construct the conditions for establishing public toilets; in other words, there was no simple cause and effect to the introduction of toilets. Most clearly, providing public toilets was forced; it was a desperate and required measure by the British government to manage the Chinese. It was made because the colonial government could not continue to ignore the urgent need for toilets.

Crucially, toilets were provided by the colonial government to further its own interests. When the health of Chinese and Europeans, especially garrisons, were linked, there were worries over an epidemic and disorder. This drove the provision to serve the government's interests. As such, the public toilet regime that was developed facilitated regulating lower-class Chinese who were believed to be producers of disease and was perceived to be an immediate solution to improving the environment in the quarter. The public toilet as moral space was a particular focus, which was seen to mediate the relationship between these Chinese and urban space; the palpable presence of morality in the daily operation of the toilets is discussed in Chap. 5. Chadwick emphasized in his report that "public latrines are most valuable means of sanitation. They should be acquired by Government, improved, their number increased, and they should be thrown open to the public gratis".[68] Under this logic, there should have been a large increase in the numbers of toilets provided by the government at public expense. However, his suggestion that there should be a large increase in public funds and land used was certainly not appreciated by the government.[69] Sanitation infrastructure, occupying land and emitting odor, was entangled with land interests, making selecting a site acceptable to all parties a difficult challenge. The development of government toilets was slow in terms of number, and less than 15 (comprising 173 seats, 25% of the total seats) were established in Victoria City by the end of the nineteenth century.[70]

Existing scholarship investigating limited government intervention in providing public toilets has focused on a variety of factors: fiscal constraints,[71] technical problems (unsophisticated drainage systems and water scarcity),[72] social tensions (objections about miasma from toilets would cause disease or depreciate property value),[73] and political conflicts (stemming from intervening in locals' daily life in colonial societies).[74] What has been missed is that the regulation of urban space in capitalist colonies such as Hong Kong was always complicated by the capitalist mode of urbanization; such changes created new power relations that were a mixture of capitalist, colonial, and ethnic forces. As public health proposals involved tensions of land revenue to the government and landowners (both Chinese and European), which led to multiple class divisions within Chinese, European and the government, they were often rejected. Therefore, the stage for the capitalist turn of sanitation infrastructure was formed in the following manner.

3.4 Competing Moral Discourses of Urban Hygiene

The capitalist dynamics, residing in the tension between regulation and profit accumulation of urban space, can be seen in the new competing discourse of urban hygiene that challenged colonial moral geography. Interlaid by race and class, it is interesting to see the multiple class divisions that came into play over sanitation policy, which shows land interest put the government, European and Chinese landowners together, contradicting the colonizer and colonized dichotomy. The multiplicities present operated along at least three divisions: capitalist, colonial and ethnic forces. New divisions emerged amongst Chinese along divisions of class: landed, elite against non-landed and lower-class people. This is seen in the fact that Chinese landowners, jointly with Chinese politicians, acted with European landowners against the interests of lower-class Chinese. Second are divisions amongst Europeans, whereby the landed class acted against the bureaucratic class. This is seen in European landowners acting with Chinese landowners in opposing health proposals formed by the government. Third are divisions internal to the colonial government, that is, the bureaucratic class and the politicians acting against the military and the sanitarians. This is seen in Hong Kong governors, government officials, and Chinese politicians opposing disease-control proposals suggested by the garrison command and sanitarians. Furthermore, Chinese politicians competed with sanitarians and government officials to provide health facilities. To disentangle the above threads, this section discusses the divisions amongst Chinese, Europeans and finally the government to explore the contradictory views that emerged towards government health implementations up until 1866, including public toilets that were established to combat disease. The discussion below examines how these parties reacted to land interests.

3.4.1 Amongst Chinese: Landed and Elite Classes Against Lower Class Chinese

With the emergence of capitalism and a focus on the land market, landowners were integrated into the colonial economic system and so were crucial to government revenue, consolidating their structural position within the colonial context. As land value grew and more land was disproportionately controlled by a small group of Chinese landowners, those who controlled much of the land could contest the mandated usage of that land. Unsurprisingly, land was becoming particularly political, fostering a favorable context for landowners to extend their control over land use, granting them a privileged position in sanitation.[75] Tensions between the government and landowners can be seen clearly in the negotiations over public health proposals. The distinctiveness of land resources in public health is important to note, as these resources were insuperable. As such, the landowners had a privileged position to determine eligibility for health provision and its location. Landed and elite classes tended to create a connection between health proposals and the loss of land by challenging the moral role of these proposals in promoting health for lower-class Chinese. This is signified in the Chinese population's rapid rise in political and economic power, which was related to the new opportunities that arose from the rapid restructuring of the economy. Here, we see the hegemonic position of powerful landowners, especially Chinese landowners, who controlled much land, working with their European counterparts and Chinese politicians in reshaping the moral discourse of urban hygiene.

Following the joint opposition by Chinese and European landowners to the *Buildings and Nuisances Ordinance,* which would have required the provision of domestic toilets in dwellings since 1856, the Memorial of 1878 to support Li Tak Cheong's building plan was signed by all major Chinese landowners. That class divisions between landowners and their tenants were seen in response to a requirement for additional ventilation made by the government, as noted in Chap. 2. What sharpened the landowners' sensibilities was the potential loss of rental space due to the proposed ventilation requirement. The point was that "land has become extremely valuable; and in order to make it profitable as an investment, it is necessary to take advantage to the utmost of the space at command," as they argued.[76] This shows that what was in the mind of these memorialists was founded on class, in their response they share the authorities' prejudice of the living style of this class of Chinese. This is reflected in the split amongst Chinese between the landed and non-landed classes, which lacked concerns for cleanliness. Nevertheless, their argument put land interests over that of sanitation and was ultimately supported by Governor Hennessy. He cautioned his subordinates that the Memorial was signed by "intelligent and influential Chinese residents whose views with respect to such questions are entailed to the greatest weight", so in the end, the ventilation proposal was shelved.[77] This is unsurprising given the structural importance of land revenue and Chinese landowners to the colony.

Landowners tended to oppose any health proposal, while the state of sanitation in the Chinese quarter continued to worsen since the 1850s. Between 1878 and 1885, deaths among Chinese individuals due to disease were high. There were least a thousand deaths from disease a year, peaking at 1,604 deaths in 1885, of a total Chinese population of 150,690 and 210,995 in 1881 and 1891, respectively.[78] The high death rate in the 1880s started a new wave of awareness about sanitation within the government. It was against such a background that the Sanitary Board submitted the *Public Health Bill* to the Colonial Secretary again in December 1886; in fact, the bill was drafted soon after the establishment of the Board in 1883, although nothing was accomplished.[79] The *Public Health Bill* stipulated domestic toilets to be included in newly constructed dwellings and further required them to be paved with hard tiles or concrete and have windows that opened to the outside. Such ambition was deftly challenged. Compared to the 1856 and 1878 Memorials, this effort reflected not only the fact that the Chinese had a deep vested interest in estate property investment but also that they began to use their links with the leading Chinese Sanitary Board member and later Legislative Councilor, Ho Kai, who voted against the Ordinance. The class division within Chinese over sanitation is well reflected in this incident. When their land interests were under threat, Chinese landowners blocked health improvements, exploiting the welfare of lower-class Chinese. Wealthy Chinese, with home buckets and access to the more hygienic public toilets in restaurants, therefore frequently sought to organize Memorials against the provision of government public toilets for lower-class Chinese, which they regarded as a sacrifice and a deprecation of land value.

The grounds behind Ho Kai's objection to the *Public Health Bill* are highlighted by his biographer G. H. Choa, who notes Ho did not see why so much land should be sacrificed for improving welfare.[80] Similarly, Ho Kai was seen by his European counterparts as exclusively looking out for landowners' interests over general sanitation.[81] We do not know the scale that he was involved in the property market, but it is certain that his father Rev. Ho Fuk Tong was a large landowner whose widow surnamed Lai was one of the top twenty taxpayers in 1881.[82] Interestingly, before the Sanitary Board submitted the *Public Health Bill* to the Colonial Secretary on 22 December 1886, Ho Kai sent a petition letter (dated December 1886) to the Colonial Secretary opposing the bill. He challenged the rationale behind the moral discourse of urban hygiene on the grounds it was based on Western sanitary science and overlooked the economic reality of Hong Kong. He argued that the even higher development costs of the measures in the bill would ultimately undermine the welfare of lower-class Chinese. Overall, as a Western medicine doctor trained in Britain and a politician appointed by the government, he severely opposed the compulsory toilet provision in dwellings proposed in the *Public Health Bill*, stating:

> Some Sanitarians are constantly making the mistake of treating Chinese as if they were Europeans…They do not allow for the differences of habits, usage, mode of living…One might as well insist that all Chinese should eat bread and beefsteak instead of rice and pork…From an economical point of view, the idea of sacrificing the millions of square feet at an average price of $6 to $7, per square foot is even more ridiculous. What is this enforced sacrifice for? Simply for the sake of a theory that the Chinese public requires all such sanitary

> improvements to promote their health and welfare. However, I challenge the soundness of that theory…It is not for the welfare of the poor to have the valuable space occupied by their small rooms narrowed, in order to have for a model of a privy…While the wicked landlords continue to charge the same rent or even a higher one for improvements and increased capital necessary to effect such improvements…all landlords, like everybody else, will want to get from 7 to 8,% net interest on their capital.[83]

Ho Kai used Western breakfast iconography, bread and beefsteak to elaborate that British habits, usage, and mode of living were incompatible with Chinese culture. This implies that the health proposals proposed by the government truly signified British cultural imperialism rather than a practice that would benefit lower-class Chinese. His argument centered on the sacrifices of the Chinese landed class and speculated about what improvements to welfare that the lower class might enjoy in the end. In his opinion, the tenants would be forced to pay higher rents for less space. He asked the government, was a 3/6 feet brick privy and spacious kitchen more necessary than food and clothing, or more desirable than overcrowding?[84] More importantly, in his opinion, the bill interfered with the interests of landowners and would shake public confidence in *laissez faire*; land investors who had benefitted from urbanization would be compelled to sacrifice their private interests for the public interest. He retained that for the benefit of Hong Kong, where economic development was highly dependent on private investment, the public interest should not be placed above private interests.

After the first reading of the *Public Health Bill* in the Legislative Council on 6 May 1887, Ho Kai started his second round of petitioning. He initiated a deputation of Chinese elites, such as Leung on, Wei Yuk and Wong Shing, to discuss the *bill* with the Acting Governor and Major General Cameron on 11 May.[85] His arguments were similar to those stated in the first petition. With the support of Ho Kai, before the second reading, a Memorial was signed by Chinese and European landowners, including the clergies of different denominations and missionary societies.[86] It is said that 47,000 Chinese people signed the Memorial.[87] It is no surprise then that the bill was passed in a modified form, with the compulsory requirement for a brick paved privy in newly constructed dwellings removed.[88] This once again shows how colonial rationalities concerning public health came into conflict with capitalist urbanization. As the colony was so deeply embedded in land-centred capitalism, health proposals were not purely a matter of sanitary science; rather, the government had to take into account private interests when attempting to implement a sound sanitation strategy for the colony.[89]

Under pressure from Chinese politicians and landowners (both Chinese and European), legislation for domestic toilets was not strictly enforced, which made the need for public toilets more urgent. Logically, the absence of domestic toilets could be compensated for through the adequate provision of public toilets. As a dedicated structure, the night soil lying in public toilet pails for hours was difficult to hide from public noses, and they were seen to deteriorate the value of surrounding properties; hence, public toilets were not a welcome solution. Interestingly, the complaints appeared not from the general Chinese community but from Chinese and European landowners. The landowners of adjacent lots always rejected government public toilet proposals on the grounds that toilet gas harmed residents and depreciated property values. Not surprisingly, competition from free-to-use government toilets was also not welcomed by the owners of privately owned toilets.[90] The rejections originated from the threat to economic interests rather than any genuine public feeling on the cleanliness of government toilets. It is true that toilet site negotiations between the government and landowners were a major obstacle to public toilet construction. It is hence easy to understand why government toilets were inadequately provided. If they were provided, they would always be located within a block of government bathhouses and markets to solve the difficulties of finding appropriate sites.[91]

Rather than campaigning for public toilets, Chinese landowners tended to use their links with politicians, for example, Ho Kai, who voted against government toilet sites and lobbied for the maintenance of the home bucket system. In one case in 1887, regarding the Sanitary Board proposal to build a public toilet at the junction of Des Voeux Street Central and Wing Lok Street (around modern-day 70 Des Voeux Street Central), Ho Kai argued there was no need to have public toilets if tenements were fully equipped with night soil buckets and urinal jars.[92] It is unclear whether his opposition to this toilet was influenced by prominent landowner Choy Chan, who owned a public toilet at 116 of the same street.[93] Seeing the sanitary problem caused by the insufficient number of government public toilets, in 1890, the government appointed a small committee of three members (Ho Kai, O. Chadwick and S. Brown, the Sanitary Board president) to investigate whether existing privately owned toilets should either be allowed to be kept by private persons for their own profit through the licensing system or whether public toilets should exclusively be under government control.[94] From the late 1860s, when the number of privately owned toilets significantly increased, the government had no power to prohibit any person who paid 60 cents per seat per month from establishing a public toilet, and worse still, it could not intervene in the charges, location or sanitary condition.[95]

Far before the 1890 report was finalized, Ho Kai openly expressed support for privately owned toilets in the Legislative Council by claiming that many landowners were eager to enter the toilet market, so there was no reason for the government to build them at public expense.[96] Moreover, he added that the toilet operators could be prosecuted if their toilets were in bad condition, which would help to keep them their facilities in a proper and sanitary order. He further argued that the sanitation provided by government toilets was no better than that provided by private toilets, so they would be an equal public nuisance in a later Sanitary Board meeting.[97] Ho Kai did not see government toilets, which were clean and a solution to poor health, as the morally charged spaces they truly were; instead, he considered their sanitary condition to be as poor as private ones. Indeed, the sanitary condition of government toilets was also a public nuisance, as seen in an 1899 report that stated they were offensive, which will be discussed in Chap. 5.[98] Three years earlier in 1887, however, as mentioned earlier, Ho Kai argued that there was no need for public toilets if night soil buckets and urinal jars were provided in tenement houses. The new contradictory argument made by him underlined the fact that the public health agenda was manipulated by landowners concerned with investment returns on their tenement housing. Therefore, the nineteenth century public toilets became a negotiated space between the government, business and elites, sanitation and profit.

The colonial surgeon sternly disagreed with Ho Kai, and he quickly rebutted that there was a great difference between the two types of toilets; government surgeons worked for the public interest, not for private interests.[99] In 1887, as mentioned earlier, Ho Kai argued that there was no need for public toilets (whether privately owned or government owned) if adequate night soil buckets were provided in dwellings. His contradictory arguments underline the fact that the public health agenda was manipulated by politicians and landowners through different interpretations of the urban hygiene discourse to fit their own interests. As land was an attractive point of investment, landowners contested with the government for the control of urban space when their land interests were under threat. Soon after Ho Kai's speech in the Legislative Council, there came an unexpected outcome: in 1888, Chinese landowners began pulling down buildings that needed to be renovated under the 1887 *Public Health Ordinance* and converted the buildings into privately owned toilets instead, with the hope of letting them to the highest bidders.[100] The landowners adopted strategies to avoid the domestic toilet requirement and then managed to turn the situation to their economic and political advantage. Their approach to sanitation rested simply on economics; toilets were perceived as a means of production. The number of conversion applications grew quickly, with over 20 in 1891 and 1892.[101] This urban contest exposed a series of underlying tensions between the government and landowners, which put the government in a very disadvantaged position. It had no power to interfere in the construction or running of privately owned toilets.

Owing to the distinctive nature of commercially oriented public pail toilets and the property development fervor that resulted from the high night soil price, the government started to examine additional necessary powers to be conferred to the Sanitary Board by legislation.[102] In such a situation, in November 1890, a by-law made under the *1887 Public Health Ordinance* was urgently enacted, empowering the government to licence and regulate the sanitary condition of privately owned public toilets.[103] The by-law established basic maintenance standards and stipulated that every public toilet building should have at least one attendant, the floors, seats and utensils should be thoroughly scrubbed at least daily, and deodorants should be used. Subsequently, the Sanitary Board passed a motion that no person should open a public toilet for the use of the public without its previous sanction.[104] Even though the toilet industry was now more regulated, toilet mania did not stop. The potential profit of toiles was too attractive to disinterest the Chinese landowners from turning their properties into toilets. They only hastened to become involved in the toilet market. Urban hygiene was then said to be captured by both the landowners, who were only concerned with economic interests, and government officials, who were mercantilists, as stated in a note made by a newspaper:

> There has lately sprung up amongst a number of Chinese landlords, some of whom are wealthy men connected with both Government and mercantile offices, a mania to pull down houses which might be in need of repair for an immediate tenant, and erect in their places latrines, which are let and sub-let to the highest bidder...are to pay these landlords from fifteen to twenty percent better than their house properties did...permission having been

granted by the Surveyor-General for the erection of fifteen…whilst plans and specifications of seven others are now being prepared… A charge of from one to two [Chinese copper] cash is made and at that rate we understand an ample profit is made.[105]

More specifically, toilet mania is well reflected in a case from August 1891, where John Lemm, an architect, applied five clients to build six toilets.[106] According to the minutes of the Sanitary Board meeting, at least sixteen applications were received throughout 1891.[107] Due to objections from neighbourhood residents, six applications to construct privately owned toilets were rejected by the Board.[108] It is not clear whether these objections came from genuine residents, general landowners or toilet landowners who were concerned about competition at their own privately owned toilets. We should note, however, that Chinese landowners split themselves into camps during this toilet mania. That toilet landowners who strongly opposed the *1887 Public Health Ordinance* remained silent during this boom in the public toilet market, showing no support to their fellow landowners. The existing toilet landowners were the principal beneficiaries of the passage of the above ordinance, as the legal status of their toilets was legitimatized, an incidental reward for their silence. Furthermore, no new privately owned toilets could be erected without the written sanction of the Sanitary Board. For the landowners, the result was somewhat like an oligopoly of the privately owned toilet market. New competitors were nearly barred by the government; only three out of sixteen applications for erecting privately owned toilets were approved in 1891.[109] In a sense, the ordinance served to reconfirm the converging interests of the government and existing toilet landowners. As such, it stands as an important sign of collaboration that legitimized both interests in the public toilet market.

In the above, we see class (landed or elite) playing an active role in shaping the provision of domestic toilets and government public toilets, determining where public toilets should be located, the condition in which they should be maintained, and who were eligible to use them. This shows that the landed and elite classes of Chinese argued that better toilet conditions would benefit lower-class Chinese; rather, they had a particular concern with private interests, specifically those of land. The reason behind this was that in terms of hygiene, they saw no difference between government and privately owned toilets. Given that both were unpleasant, the private ones were just as useful to solving the sanitary problem posed by lower-class Chinese relieving themselves in public, simply by shifting the problem to inside the toilets. Obviously, landowners did not share authorities' concerns over the moral role of toilets in maintaining urban hygiene. They did not consider public toilets as a morally charged space that could induce sanitary habits in Chinese; rather, they saw toilets as a technology to capture night soil as a means of production. It is clear that those with huge land resources played a decisive role in urban hygiene, challenging colonial moral geography.

It is essential to grasp one fundamental point: the challenges to urban land use posed by landowners indicate how land resources allowed them to reshape policies in favor of their own class interests. This suggests a class for itself: this class was realized in the contests over the use of urban space, which has a key role in the arising of consciousness.[110] They came to feel a group identity born of shared interests, which worked against the interests of lower-class Chinese. Challenges by Chinese landed and elites against the government were very visible, and these challenges were prompted by the government intervening in toilet economies in a mission to improve the sanitary conditions of lower-class Chinese. Unsurprisingly, land had become particularly political in the land capitalist context, and those in possession of such land could often reshape public health logic during the contest with the government.[111]

3.4.2 *Amongst Europeans: Landed Class and Elite Classes Against the Bureaucratic Class*

Chinese landowners were not alone in challenging the potential role of public toilets in the colony's hygiene. Unsurprisingly, tensions between land profits and spatial regulation were also found between European landowners and the government. As has already been seen, European landowners sided with their Chinese counterparts to oppose the domestic toilet proposals in 1856 and 1887. With the vibrant land market, urban space became a marketable product, and internal divisions between landed European capitalists and the bureaucrat class over sanitation were unavoidable. For example, H. Ruttonjee, father of J. H. Ruttonjee who was the founder of Ruttonjee Hospital, argued that a proposed public toilet at Elgin Road in Kowloon would cause unpleasantness to his newly built hotel across the road.[112] As a consequence, the proposed toilet was abandoned. Similarly, the Land Investment Company objected to a toilet at Gillies Avenue in Kowloon.[113] The reason behind this objection was that it would depreciate the value of a nearby property. The Sanitary Board, then, shifted the proposed site a short distance; however, the company objected again. In response, the Colonial Secretary argued in a letter that if the owner would provide toilets in the houses, the erection of public toilets might not be necessary. Like other landowners keen on pursing land interests, the company argued it was undesirable to put toilets among a better class of houses and that a toilet would depreciate the value of houses. Therefore, it suggested a site, however it was approximately 300 m away from a considerable aggregation of houses that the toilet was intended to serve. This time the Board did not compromise and insisted on the original site, the proposal was passed in the Legislative Council with the support of the Governor in the Executive Council.

Another example is the British press criticizing government officials, describing them as "mercantilists"[114] who colluded with toilet landowners and encouraged the 1891 toilet mania. The press publicly wondered why the discussion of licensing of privately owned toilets, which started in 1890, ended abruptly in early 1891. The papers argued that part of the reason was that the Sanitary Board was toothless and partly that the "mercantile" Surveyor General only approved the erection of privately owned toilets because he wanted to maintain a good relationship with the Chinese who would contribute tax, so he did not undertake his responsibility of maintaining sanitation in the colony. At the end of the commentary, the editor desperately stated,

> In the absence of such bodies [as a Municipal Council or urban authority], we can only look forward to that body [the Sanitary Board], which is responsible for existing evils, and should further evils spring up they ought to be laid at the door of those whose duty it is, but who fail to us the proper means of prevention.[115]

In the conflicts between landed and government Europeans, we first see that objections to government toilets were linked to land interests. Capital accumulation at the expense of urban hygiene crossed the racial divide, uniting the aspirations of European and Chinese landowners. Such a complex situation crossed ethnic borders, meaning new alliances were created between elite Europeans and Chinese in opposing health proposals, against the wishes and best outcomes for the colonial government, the local garrison, and lower-class Chinese. Second, the British press publicly argued that the powerlessness and the apparent mercantilism of the authorities in regulating privately owned toilets was a consequence of a political compromise on the economic forces of Chinese landowners. This implied that the morality of government officials did not always conform to the Western standard (concerning public health) when faced with economic interests.

3.4.3 Amongst the Government: Military and Sanitarians Against Governors, Officials, and Chinese Politicians

The colonial government itself was by no means the only part of the government system in which politicians, sanitarians, military officials and the colonial office had a say. When toilet provision was entangled with land interests in the land-based revenue system, the government itself was split based on what they perceived the public interest to be—sanitation or land revenue. The military and the Sanitary Board, for example, frequently advocated for public health improvement, but the Governor Hennessy and those from Public Works looked at revenue. We have seen the division between Chinese Sanitary Board members and the Legislative Councillors Ho Kai and Wei Yuk and their European counterparts over the provision of domestic toilets required in 1887. Here, we move to the division between the Director of the Public Works Department and members of the Sanitary Board and between the Governor and the Surgeon General of Army Medical Department.

It is important here to keep in mind the great difficulties in improving urban hygiene due to high land prices, which Chadwick had seen in his short stay in Hong Kong in the 1880s. He observed that "I am aware that the great cost of land does not give much opportunity for so doing".[116] Therefore, he suggested having more government toilets and put them in open space to encourage better air circulation. In response to the proposal for a toilet in Gough Street in the 1900s, it was cancelled after the Public Works Department complained about the loss of land revenue, as noted in Chap. 1. Following the failure of this proposal, another site was located at the junction of Des Voeux Road West and Connaught Road West, and a proposal for this site submitted by the Board was also turned down.[117] The Director of the Department, W. Chatham, stated he was not in favor of placing such a structure on a main road because they were more expensive to maintain there, and the Department had insufficient funding to do so. It is obvious that the department did not have the budget for toilet, which made the Director more concerned with land value than urban hygiene. This is also reflected in an official record that shows that a cheap resumption cost, rather than the needs of the community, was the decisive factor for when the Director approved a toilet site.

As the land in the most prosperous part of Victoria City had already been fully occupied, there was no more open space upon which public toilets in the most convenient locations for users could be erected. It was therefore necessary to find a suitable, affordable site for resumption. Since houses in Chuk Hing Lane were valued at HK$2,842, much cheaper than another proposed site in Tung Tak Lane at HK$14,911, Chuk Hing Lane was chosen.[118] As the value of land fluctuated, the resumption cost increased to HK$300 per toilet seat (total 16 seats), for a total of approximately HK$5,000.[119] However, as a government official, the director was obliged to support the resumption out of the department budget, and he showed reluctance, saying that "it seems to me it would become a very serious task to provide accommodation to anything like the extent it [public toilets] ought to be provided throughout the city".[120] At the same meeting, two prominent Chinese councilors, Ho Kai and Wei Yuk, objected, arguing that Chuk Hing Lane was a bad site. They argued that the site was surrounded by the back of houses three stories high and would have a significant effect on the kitchens of the adjacent houses. Ho Kai argued there were contradictions in the government moral discourse of urban hygiene; on the first hand, the government had called on landowners to put in more windows to allow further fresh air, but on the other hand, it compelled tenants to open those windows and so admit foul air stemming from the toilets in the immediate vicinity. In response to Ho's opposition, the Colonial Secretary H. May argued that he did not see sufficient grounds to block the proposed toilet from being constructed; he said that "there are a great many latrines in the city of Victoria…and every one of them is theoretically open to the very same objection that the senior unofficial member [Ho Kai] has urged against this particular one".[121] There could be only one answer: the vested interests in property development. In the end, the proposal was passed two years after it was proposed.[122]

There was also apparent disagreement between the Public Works Department and other government officials over who should pay for sanitation and the associated public toilet scheme. In an earlier Sanitary Board meeting in 1891, the Registrar General seized the opportunity to condemn the Department to ignore the impact of public toilets on the surrounding environment.[123] The argument began from J. Cantile, the founding Dean of the Hong Kong College of Medicine and a teacher of Sun Yat Sen (the national father of China) who complained a privately owned toilet established immediately opposite to the teaching hospital, Alice Memorial Hospital, would cause a nuisance to patients. The hospital, its formation spearheaded by Ho Kai in 1887, served as the teaching hospital of the college.[124] The Registrar General seized this objection to support his more general contention that no place ought to be used for a public toilet without a licence from the Sanitary Board. He criticized that the department was an irresponsible toilet landowner for having built a public toilet opposite a church years ago. He pointed out that mistakes in the selection of suitable locations were due to the department acting independently and proudly claimed that the board would be less likely to make such mistakes. The Registrar General made the severe comment that department officials were "sinners", as business ends seemed to characterize their morality, and this was as low as that of Chinese business, which aimed to keep toilets an object of business speculation.

Nevertheless, privately owned toilets were both a means of production and a sanitation infrastructure, and as a member of the committee aimed to discuss the licensing of privately owned toilets shown earlier, Chadwick changed his mind and supported these toilets in 1890.[125] Not long before, in 1882, Chadwick was still insisting that public toilets were a moral space that exercised moral governance on Chinese and so should be put in the hands of the government. As seen in the first section, Chadwick also clearly understood the difficulty in providing government toilets in a land capitalist context, so the reality compelled him to support the privately owned offerings given the insufficient number of toilets overall. This was an important and dramatic change because it shows that sanitarians such as Chadwick were very worried about the general sanitary condition of the colony and thus adopted a pragmatic view towards privately owned toilets. In a sense, this echoed what Ho Kai argued earlier, that sanitary science alone could not bring about sanitation improvements; rather, there needed to be an emphasis on private interest. In this case, the blending of private and public concerns in public toilets was an eclectic way to improve general colony sanitation. This might explain why the Sanitary Board and the Surveyor General tended to approve the provision of privately owned toilets while imposing regulations on their sanitary condition.

Owing to the capitalist context, health-related proposals could not be easily implemented. Amongst the governors, Hennessy was the one most criticized for compromising public health (e.g., rejecting the public toilet provision to avoid sacrificing land for development) for better relations with the Chinese elites, who were the main taxpayers and had a deep vested interest in land development that meant they continually opposed such implementations. In the first section, we saw the arguments between Hennessy and the military about the sanitary condition of Chinese houses, which stemmed from the relaxation of restrictions upon Chinese purchasing houses in European areas. Here, we focus on his support for the traditional Chinese home bucket system and challenge to the flush toilet system, which was regarded by his European contemporaries as the solution to poor public health. Endacott explains that Hennessy ignored public health because his "respect for Chinese customs and interests blinded him to the danger of the sanitary condition".[126] His objection to a flush toilet proposal aroused much argument amongst the government, mainly from the military and sanitarians. Speaking from cultural and ecological perspectives, Hennessy argued his support for the bucket system that,

> Having here a native population who will readily carry out the Chinese custom by which the sewage and refuse is carried out of the town, and used for agricultural purposes. Having a population accustomed to that sensible practice, I have very little doubt this colony can be made a model of sanitation…Professor Huxley said that some Oriental nations, that we had been in the habit of calling barbarous, were actually more civilized than ourselves in the mode in which they treat sewage.[127]

Hennessy's high-profile support for the bucket system, by which the waste was used for agricultural purposes, was seen by him to be more civilized than a flush toilet system, which had a high danger of infection due to the unsophisticated drainage of the time. He was severely critical of flush toilets, towards which he mocked the so-called "Western sanitary science."[128] He pointed out that in Britain, the primary sanitary problem was the proper disposal of sewer water and that sewers facilitated the transference of miasma and organic molecules from house to house and place to place. As the pipes may occasionally burst or leak, the ground could be contaminated, and consequently, the water supply was in constant danger. Hennessy believed that the dangers of sewage were greater when concealed underground and out of individual control. Rather, he saw that a pail system meant that China and Hong Kong were entirely free of the danger of disease moving from house to house through sanitation piping. Therefore, he suggested that the bucket system, with the added procedure of applying a layer of dry earth to night soil, could minimize miasma far better than a flush system, improving general sanitation. His support for the bucket system and the rejection of the flush system obviously contrasted with some of his European contemporaries, and not surprisingly, this led to complaints. The most influential complaint was made by the Surgeon General of Army Medical Department in Britain, W. A. Mackinnon, who severely criticized Hennessy after observing sanitary matters in Hong Kong in 1881. He stated, "There has been a complete reversal of the wise policy of his predecessors in sanitary matters…his Excellency has derived his inspirations from ignorant Chinese traders, and trading guilds composed of unscientific natives".[129] Mackinnon's complaint about Hennessy immediately led to Chadwick being dispatched by the colonial office to investigate the sanitary condition of the colony.

Hennessy embellished the advantages of the bucket system while overlooking the difficulties that it posed in a densely populated city such as Victoria City. At the same time, he was correct to point out the issues with the current implementations of the flush system. Today, we are used to the toilet flush system as an effective means of disease control, so we are likely to question whether Hennessy's opposition to flush toilets was due to a political compromise with Chinese business. However, contemporary assumptions also embellish colonial powers' achievement of hygienic modernity and the success of flush systems in the nineteenth century. For example, is Leicester in 1895, located in the East Midlands of Britain, which only had 13,000 flush toilets, the city remained highly dependent upon 6,700 pails.[130] Factors such as the scarcity of water, a costly and unsophisticated sewage system, and sewage pollution to rivers contributed to the limited use of a flush system. In the words of Wohl, a British public health historian, there is an illusion of how pervasive the system was in the nineteenth century:

> Public health historians, perhaps focusing too narrowly on the splendid creation in the 1860s of a system of main sewers in London…Primitive and defective privies and the dry conservancy methods of disposal continued to exist down to the end of the century, and at the end of Queen Victoria's reign w.cs were still unknown to the majority of her subjects.[131]

It can be said that the very colonial idea of a neat structural boundary between modern and traditional, East and West, in social and technical development is too simple. Differing little from the colonies, urban hygiene in Europe was mainly sustained using the pail system and the traditional practice of night soil disposal. However, pail and flush systems were put partially into practice in the 1820s and 1850s in Britain, respectively.[132] Flush systems did not become common until the early twentieth century.[133] In the nineteenth century, there were frequent charges made against the flush system, that it was not well formulated, that stagnant decomposition took place, and that drains were ineffective at trapping any gas, which prevented flow back due to technical problems.[134] Most problematic, however, was that harbors and rivers came to serve as extended cesspools. Sewer waste was flushed into rivers—the Port Hamburg of Germany, the Mississippi of the United States and the Thames of Britain—and the water quality from these sewage-contaminated rivers was poor.[135] The flushing of sewage into waterways greatly increased the chance of infection, and so at the time for the flush system, the connections between disease, sewage and water were greater than for the pail system.[136] This worry about contamination was illustrated in the writings of Edwin Chadwick: "The whole of the modern system of sewage and water-closets is blamed, and a return to the old system of cesspits talked of and earth closets proposed as substitutes".[137] Sanitarians hesitated to endorse the flush system and rather expressed the view that the pail system was preferable.

These critical views about flush toilet systems were carried to Hong Kong, and the government even fined the owners of houses that were connected to the main sewers, as per the 1856 *Buildings and Nuisances Ordinance*.[138] By 1880, there were 182 water closets, mainly situated in European company premises, homes and hotels, but these were truly water commodes (which can be seen as a simple form of septic tank) that were not connected to the city's main sewers.[139] In this regard, the Surveyor General and Inspector of Buildings shared Hennessy's opposition to the flush system, the latter claimed he would not support such a system even with sufficient water supply due to the potential miasma that could stem from the sewers.[140] In a similar manner, Chadwick did not recommend the use of the flush system in public toilets; rather, he suggested an improved form of pail system with better toilet and facility designs (e.g., more windows, boat-shaped vessels) and polished materials (earthware or cast iron) to increase ventilation and minimize dirt accumulation.[141] In this discussion, I have no intention to fight the assertion that Hennessy's support for the bucket system was aimed at maintaining a good relationship with the Chinese. Rather, I place debates on the merits and demerits of a flush toilet system into its historical context to unravel the class politics that occurred within government. This discussion also displays how weak the boundary between the modern West and traditional East truly was at the time and so how the internal politics within the colonial government often pierced this boundary too.

These multiple internal divisions of class arose over the moral discourse of urban hygiene and how to maintain colony health. They are crucial to understanding how critical land revenue and resources were in determining public health policies, specifically the public toilet initiative in early colonial Hong Kong. If land interests were so important, what new spatial order, manifested by the capitalist system, would appear out of the colonial order (that was derived from a discursive moral order of Otherness)? There are four crucial points to note about contestation over hygiene moral discourse. First, domestic and public types of toilets that would both undermine land profit were seen to be unnecessary provisions. This assertion rejected the government's claim that toilets were the solution to poor general health and their potential moral role in regulating the relationship between bodily habits and urban space. Second, toilet provision became entangled with land interests in the land-based revenue system, which always hemmed the government in a land market agenda when regulating space. This is well reflected in the divisions that occurred between the Sanitary Board and the Public Works Department over toilet provision and location. This is a tension between rational regulation and profit accumulation of urban space.

Third was the negotiation of space between the government and the Chinese elites. The contestation of local business (in alliance with Chinese politicians) over the use of urban space was integrated with the new opportunities that were arising because of the capitalist restructuring of the economy. This is shown in the rapid rise of Chinese elite political and economic capital, which meant they felt confident enough to challenge the government's moralizing discourse of the toilet. This indicates that morality alone was not enough to regulate urban space, so proponents of the moral argument needed to take into account the business's land interests. Fourth, this not only meant that public health services were to not necessarily be provided by the government but also indicated that there was no inevitable contradiction between capitalist and moralist interests and that the public toilet as a means of production could successfully embody both interests.

3.5 Conclusion

Underlying the public toilet project was a fear of disease that might originate from lower-class Chinese and Chinese quarters. Chinese people were perceived by the government as a major factor causing the high mortality of Europeans and garrisons. This connection alarmed the government, making them hope to improve sanitation through public toilets. However, colonial urban order came to be mediated by the market through the process of capitalist urbanization. This created a dilemma of governing urban space in a land capitalist reality but also opened opportunities in nineteenth-century Hong Kong. It was within the government-capitalist dynamic that multiple internal class divisions over sanitation existed, in contrast to the dichotomy of colonizer and colonized. This revealed a tangle of land interests, setting the stage for the capitalist turn of sanitation. The interference of the land market complicated the workings of colonial administration, creating the conditions for the restructuring of colonial urban order, which opened new opportunities for colonial collaboration over public toilet provision, blending moral and economic logics.

Notes

1. Ord 24 of 87: Public Health, CO129/234, 1 Nov 1887, p. 126–7. Cameron was acting between April and October 1887.
2. Laws relating to Public Health, *GG*, 23 July 1887, p. 875.
3. Cowell, 2013; Endacott, 1964; Munn, 2009.
4. Eitel, 1895: 191.
5. Lau, 2002: 8.
6. Great Morality among the Troops, CO129/17, 19 August 1846, p. 92–102; To the Editor of the Friend of China, *FoC*, 30 November 1843.
7. Evans, 1970; Yip, 2009.
8. Cowell. 2013: 359.
9. Removal of Public Privy, CO129/10, 20 October 1843, p. 521–2.
10. Commentaries, *FoC*, 1 June and 31 July 1844. Improvement of the Colony, CO129/10, 26 December 1844, p. 310–22.
11. To the Editor of the Friend of China, *FoC*, 30 November 1843; Commentaries, *FoC*, 3 August 1844.
12. Pomfret, 2013; Swanson, 1977.
13. Cowell, 2013; Evans, 1970; Munn, 2009.
14. An Ordinance for the Preservation of Good Order and Cleanliness, GG, 20 March 1844, No. 5 of 1844. https://www.oelawhk.lib.hku.hk/archive/files/2b4c38ded8e441159b4dcb8f05f1073d.pdf. (accessed 17 December 2020).
15. Commentaries, *FoC*, 7 August 1844; Evans, 1970.
16. Manderson, 1996; Pomfret, 2013.
17. Arnold, 1994; Yeoh, 1996; Swanson, 1977.
18. *FoC*, 4 May 1844; Smith, 1985: 45–7.
19. Chan, 1991; Hui, 1996; Sinn, 2003.
20. Carroll, 2007; Munn, 2009.
21. Population, *BB*, 1871, 1881, 1891.
22. Ibid, 1911.
23. Ibid, 1901, 1921.
24. Chadwick, 1882: 11.
25. Annual Report of the Colonial Surgeon for 1879, 4 May 1880. Sanitary Reports, *AR*, 1880.
26. Chapman, 1971; Wohl, 1983.
27. Letter from Colonial Surgeon to the Acting Colonial Secretary, 1875. Sanitary Reports, *AR*, 1880.
28. Report of the Colonial Surgeon on his Inspection of the Town of Victoria, 15 April 1874. Sanitary reports, *AR*, 1880.
29. Letter from Colonial Surgeon to Acting Colonial Secretary, 28 July 1880. Sanitary Reports, *AR*, 1880.

30. Reports of the Medical Officer of Health, the Sanitary Surveyor, and the Colonial Veterinary Surgeon for the Year 1897, *SP*, 1898, p. 270.
31. Chadwick, 1882; Eitel, 1895.
32. Public Health and Housing, *The Lancet*, 2 March 1901, p. 604; Wohl, 1983.
33. Population, *BB*, 1891, p. 373.
34. Wohl, 1983.
35. Letter from Colonial Surgeon to Acting Colonial Secretary, 28 July 1880. Sanitary Reports, *AR*, 1880. More about Chinese living style, see Report of the Colonial Surgeon on his Inspection of the Town of Victoria, 15 April 1874. Sanitary Report, *AR*, 1880; Yellow Fever, *GG*, 12 May 1866, p. 190.
36. Chapman, 1971; Wohl, 1983.
37. Chadwick, 1882: 19; Colonial Surgeon to Acting Colonial Secretary, 28 July 1880. Sanitary Reports, *AR*, 1880.
38. Report of the Licenced Brothels, 19 January 1874. Sanitary Reports, *AR*, 1880.
39. Report of the Colonial Surgeon on his Inspection of the Town of Victoria, 15 April 1874. Sanitary Reports, *AR*, 1880.
40. CSR for 1893, *GG*, 1 December 1894, p. 364.
41. CSR for 1853, *GG*, 29 April 1854, p. 358.
42. CSR for 1858, *GG*, 19 March 1859, p. 85; RCHK, Letter from Acting Assistant Military Secretary to Colonial Secretary, 22 August 1879. Enclosure 7 in No. 19, *BPP 1863–81*. Vol. 25, 1971, p. 680.
43. CSR for 1853, *GG*, 29 April 1854, p. 358.
44. Report of Colonial Surgeon, 29 August 1879. *BPP 1882–99*. Vol. 26, 1971, p. 26.
45. RCHK, Minutes by the Registrar General, 16 May 1877. Enclosure 3, in No. 1, *BPP 1863–1881*, Vol. 25, 1971, p. 651.
46. RCHK, Letter from Major-General to the Secretary for State for War, 5 February 1881. Enclosure in No. 34, *BPP* 1863–1881, Vol. 25, 1971, p. 708.
47. RCHK, Letter from Major-General to the Secretary for State for War, 14 January 1880. Enclosure 1 in No. 9, *BPP* 1863–1881, Vol. 25, 1971, p. 658–9. More about his complaint, see RCHK, Letter from Major-General to the Secretary of State for War, 20 December 1878. Enclosures in No. 3; Letter from Major-General to the Military Secretary, 6 December 1879. Enclosure in No. 6; Letter from Major-General to the Secretary of State for War, 5 February 1881. Enclosure in No. 34, *BPP* 1863–1881. Vol. 25, 1971, p. 652–709. For government revenue, see Revenue and Expenditure, *BB*, 1877.
48. RCHK, Letter from Governor to Earl of Kimberley, 8 July 1880. Enclosure in No. 19, *BPP 1863–1881*, Vol. 25, 1971, p. 665.
49. Letter from Colonial Office to War Office, 21 September 1881. Enclosure in No. 3, *BPP 1882–99*, Vol. 26, p. 27.
50. The European District Reservation Ordinance, *GG*, 24 November 1888, p. 1070.
51. Swanson, 1977: 390. See also Levin, 1998.

52. Hill District Reservation Ordinance, *GG*, 31 March 1904, p.584. See also Pomfret, 2013.
53. Wohl, 1983: 8.
54. McFarlane, 2008.
55. Mortality among the Chinese Population, *GG*, 10 May 1856, No. 58.
56. An Ordinance for Buildings and Nuisances, *GG*, 29 March 1856.
57. The Buildings and Nuisances Ordinance, *GG*, 6 December 1856, No.132. The Buildings and Nuisances Ordinance, CO129/59, 11 Novermber1856, p. 18–79. See also Endacott, 1964; Munn, 2009.
58. Yellow Fever, *GG*, 12 May 1866, No.71, p.189.
59. SCR, *GG*, 1 April 1865, p. 160; SCR, *GG*, 17 March 1866, p. 125.
60. Yellow Fever, *GG*, 12 May 1866, No.71, p.190.
61. Yellow Fever, *GG*, 12 May 1866, No.71, 193.
62. Note 13; An Ordinance to repeal Ordinance No.5 of 1844, GG, 26 December 1845. https://www.oelawhk.lib.hku.hk/archive/files/87c8a2538862dfbe6bc2c87d2e9f5179.pdf. (accessed 17 December 2020).
63. The Hong Kong Police Force, *GG*, 6 September 1862, No. 91, p. 254.
64. Yellow Fever, *GG*, 12 May 1866, p.190.
65. Observation by Surgeon General, 1 September 1880. Enclosure in No. 10, *BPP 1882–99*, Vol. 26, p. 45.
66. CRN, HKRS149-2-534, 1869; Order and Cleanliness Ordinance, *GG*, 22 June 1867, No. 96, p. 232.
67. Anderson, 1996; Macpherson, 1987; Rogaski, 2004.
68. Chadwick, 1882: 5.
69. Correspondence regarding the Sanitary Condition of Hong Kong, *SP*, 1901; Sanitation of the Colony, CO129/305, 1901, pp. 637–68.
70. *RLUA*, 1899, p. 7–12.
71. Yeoh, 1996; Macpherson, 1987; Yu, 2010.
72. Hamlin, 1988; Macpherson, 1987; Yeoh, 1996.
73. Brunton, 2005; Jackson, 2014.
74. Yeoh, 1996.
75. Chu, 2013a; Endacott, 1964.
76. Chinese Houses, *GG*, 27 July 1878, p. 371.
77. Ibid, p. 372.
78. For the death rate, see CSR for the 1885, *GG*, 26 June 1886, p. 286. For the population, see Census of Hong Kong, *GG*, 11 July 1891, No. 297, p. 549.
79. Sanitary Board's letter submitting Public Health Bill, 22 December 1886. Papers presented to Legislative Council, *SP*, 27 May 1887, p. 411–2. See also Choa, 1981.
80. Choa, 1981.
81. The Sanitary Board's Rejoinder, 1 June 1887. Papers presented to Legislative Council, *SP*, 27 May 1887, p. 407–10. More about Ho's defended landowners' interests, see Endacott, 1964; Smith, 1971.
82. His land investment from Carroll 2007: 124. Tax from AJPH, *GG*, 7 February 1882, p. 82.

83. Dr. Ho Kai's Protest, 2 December 1886. Papers presented to Legislative Council, *SP*, 27 May 1887, p. 403–7.
84. Ibid, p. 405.
85. Choa, 1981: 81.
86. Public Health Bill, *HKDP*, 6 July 1887.
87. Endacott, 1964: 201.
88. The Public Health Ordinance 1887, *GG*, 2 June 1888, No. 7, p. 531–44.
89. Choa, 1981; Endacott, 1964.
90. Latrines in Hong Kong, *HKT*, 9 February 1891.
91. Crown Property, *HKBB*, 1891–1911.
92. MSB, *GG*, 29 October 1887, No. 446, p. 1196.
93. *RB*, HKRS 38-2-57, 1887.
94. Public Latrines, *CM*, 7 March 1890; Latrines in Hong Kong, *HKT*, 9 February 1891.
95. For the limitations of government, see Public Latrines, *HKT*, 7 January 1891; Latrines in Hong Kong, *HKT*, 9 February 1891. For the tax, Schedule of Taxes, Duties, Fees, *BB*, 1882, p. A2.
96. Public Latrines, *HKH*, 5 December 1890, p. 77.
97. Public Latrines, *HKT*, 7 January 1891.
98. Hong Kong Government, 1899.
99. Public Latrines, *HKT*, 7 January 1891.
100. MSB, *GG*, 8 December 1888; Public Latrines in Hong Kong, *HKT*, 26 March 1891.
101. Public Latrine, *GG*, 7 February 1891, No. 44, p. 76; Public Latrines in Hong Kong, *HKT*, 26 March 1891; MSB, *GG*, 7 February, 22 August, 24 October, 14 November 1891, 26 December 1891.
102. MSB, *GG*, 8 December 1888; 2 February, 5 February 1889.
103. Latrines, *GG*, 21 February 1891, No. 63, p. 124.
104. MSB, *GG*, 14 March 1891.
105. Public Latrines in Hong Kong, *HKT*, 26 March 1891.
106. MSB, *GG*, 22 August, No. 362, p. 768. For more applications, see MSB, *GG*, 24 October 1891, No. 434, p. 925; and 14 November 1891, No. 457, p. 1021.
107. MSB, *GG*, 7 February, 11 July, 22 August 1891.
108. MSB, *GG*, 6 February, 5 September, 24 October, 26 December 1891.
109. MSB, *GG*, 5 September, 28 November 1891.
110. Thompson, 1983.
111. Chu, 2013a; Endacott, 1964.
112. Latrine in Elgin Road, *CM*, 13 August 1901; A Public Nuisance, *HKT*, 15 May 1900; Latrine in Elgin Road, *GG*, 10 February 1900, No. 46, p.186.
113. Latrine in Hung Hom, *HKH*, 27 February 1902, p. 3–4.
114. Public Latrines in Hong Kong, *HKT*, 26 March 1891.
115. Ibid.
116. Chadwick, 1882: 55.
117. Gough Street Latrine, *SCMP*, 18 January 1907.
118. Public Latrine in Chuk Hing Lane, *SP*, 1908, No. 999.

119. Resolution under the Public Health Ordinance, *HKH*, 18 June 1908, p. 75.
120. Ibid.
121. Resolution under the Public Health Ordinance, *HKH*, 18 June 1908, p. 75.
122. Resolution of the Legislative Council, *GG*, 19 June 1908, No. 429, p. 713.
123. Latrines in Hong Kong, *HKT*, 9 February 1891.
124. Choa, 1980.
125. Public Latrines in Hong Kong, *HKT*, 26 March 1891.
126. Endacott, 1964: 186.
127. AJPH, *GG*, 11 February 1882, p. 77.
128. Sanitary Reports, *AR*, 1880; RCHK, Letter from the Governor to the Earl of Kimberley, 8 July 1880. No. 19, *BPP 1863–81*, Vol. 25, 1971, p. 663–8; Minutes by the Governor, 28 May 1877. *BPP 1882–1899*, Vol. 26, 1971, p. 23–6.
129. Observation by Surgeon General, Enclosure in No. 10. *BPP 1882–99*, Vol. 26, 1971, p. 45.
130. Wohl, 1983: 95.
131. Ibid.
132. Brunton, 2005: 188, 192.
133. Wohl, 1983.
134. Gandy, 2006; Hamlin, 1988; Jackson, 2014.
135. Evans, 1987; Frazer, 1950; Melosi, 2000.
136. Trough Closet, *Public Health*, Vol. 7, October 1894, p. 297; Water Closets without Water, The Lancet, Vol. 149, 5 June 1897, p. 1557–8.
137. Chadwick, 1997: 638.
138. An Ordinance for Buildings and Nuisances, *GG*, 29 March 1856.
139. Water-Closets in Hong Kong, Minutes by the Governor, 3 August 1880. Annual Report of the Colonial Surgeon for 1879, *AR*, 1880.
140. Letter from Inspector of Buildings to Surveyor General, 20 August 1880. Sanitary Reports, *AR*, 1880; RCHK, Letter from Surveyor General to Acting Colonial Secretary, 30 June 1880. *BPP* 1863–81, Vol. 25, 1971, p. 713–6.
141. Chadwick, 1882.

Chapter 4
Toilet Economies: Night Soil Profit, Entrance Fees and Rent

4.1 Overview

This chapter explores the commercialization of public toilet provision (both government-owned and privately owned) in nineteenth-century Hong Kong, which was shaped by the pursuit of speculative land and night soil profits. The waste deposited in the toilets was the preferred fertilizer for Southern China's booming silk industry, tying public sanitation to global consumer markets within the world system. The author discusses the influence of the macroeconomic environment on microeconomic and public toilet developments in the colony. Land-centered capitalism and a government night soil monopoly supported the creation of market-oriented public toilets, which were a mechanism to mediate the micropolitics (especially the land and night soil interests) between the Hong Kong colonial government and Chinese business in everyday life. Toilet economies—night soil sales, entrance fees, and land rental—were critical to the economic sustainability of public toilets, especially privately owned ones, adding complexity to sanitation development and government-business relations. In the capitalist context, the toilets' primary function was the commercial collection of night soil, so they were inevitably seen as marketable public space.

The predominance of privately owned public toilets (occupied 75% of total public toilet seats) in the nineteenth century represented an important transcendence of colonizer-colonized and public–private boundaries. This symbolizes a change in the public role played by the government and private Chinese business and a change to a new set of powers and relations in the political economy of the colony. This ultimately supported a tilt towards Chinese sharing governance with the government in daily life. Throughout this, it is interesting to see that the collective goal of reordering urban space to be marketable and ordered came to be achieved through the actions and interests of government and business at such an early stage of capitalism. This raises the following question: can we develop a new model of spatial relations between government and business in urban hygiene in that toilets were transformed into marketable space and discern a wider implication for the market-oriented toilet

Y. Chong, *Toilet as Business for the Hygiene of the Chinese Community in Colonial Hong Kong*, https://doi.org/10.1007/978-981-19-1396-9_4

landscape? In the following, the author discusses the role of the key players (night soil contractors, toilet operators, toilet landowners, landowners, the governor and the administrative officials) in transforming toilets into marketable space and the impact of toilet economies.

Motivated by the rising demand for night soil in Shunde located in the Pearl River Delta from the 1860s and the potential profits in trading land, Hong Kong Chinese drove a dramatic change in the colony's public toilet landscape. The number of privately owned toilets more than tripled almost overnight, from six in 1867 to 22 a year later.[1] Throughout the boom in silk and night soil demand, the number of privately owned toilets remained high, even after the outbreaks of the plague in 1894, and most of the time remained common until the end of the nineteenth century, when night soil demand began to decline due to a combination of factors such as disasters in China and the downtrend of the global silk market (Fig. 4.1).

It was only as long as night soil profits remained attractive, which lasted until approximately 1899, that privately owned public toilets leased for higher rental as they functioned as night soil collection points remained predominant. The operation of private toilets was driven by night soil profit and land interests, which raises three important points. First, the role of private interest and Chinese were not as static as they may first appear, as they eventuated that public toilets did not necessarily need to be provided by the government and could also be provided by Chinese private enterprises. Second, toilet services were underpinned by night soil, which put the service at the mercy of business. Third, services could be operated on a quasi-commercial basis, thus blending both capitalist and moral concerns within toilet space so that a new moral geography was formed. As profits dwindled and

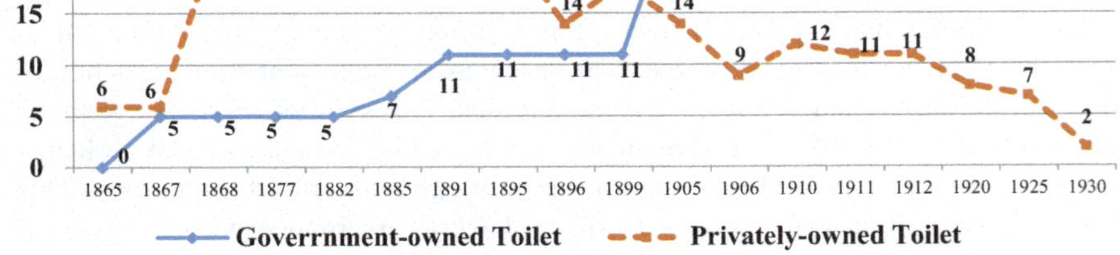

Fig. 4.1 Number of Government-owned and Privately owned Public Toilets in Victoria City, 1865–1930. *Source* The author compiled the data from the following documents: Chadwick, 1882; CRN, HKRS149-2-1247, 1885, HKRS149-2-1415, 1889; Crown Property, *BB*, 1891–1911; HKRS38-2, *RB*, 1865–1930; Hong Kong Government, 1899.
Note There were no government toilets prior to 1867. Due to data limitations, the number after 1912 is unknown

Table 4.1 Events related to the development of public toilets

Year	Event
1867	Introduction of public toilet system
1868	Great increase of privately owned public toilets
1869	Introduction of night soil tender system
1877–1882	Administration of Governor Hennessy who supported bucket system
1878–1885	High mortality of Chinese due to health crises
1887	Introduction of Public Health Ordinance
1890	Introduction of the by-law on public toilets
1894	Outbreak of plague
1897	Introduction of Latrine Ordinance
1900–1910s	Disasters in China decreased night soil demand
1915	Pirates ransom night soil contractors, causing huge losses in the night soil business
1916	Political disturbance in China caused difficulty in transporting night soil
The end of 1920s	Decline of silk industry decreased night soil demand

Sources The author compiled various sources shown in the text from various chapters

business-owned toilets were closed, there was a significant increase in the number of government toilets from the early twentieth century onwards (Table 4.1).

4.2 China's Silk Industry and the World Silk Market

The economic value of night soil was critical to the development of public toilets; therefore, it is necessary to have a basic understanding of silk production along the Pearl River Delta in Guangdong Province in the nineteenth and early twentieth centuries. China's silk industry was opened to the world after the First Opium War and the establishment of the five treaty ports of Fuzhou, Guangzhou, Ningbo, Shanghai, and Xiamen under the Treaty of Nanking, 26 June 1843.[2] First, a region near Shanghai was the primary silk production area in China. Situated at the mouth of the Yangtze River and beside a deep-water harbour, Shanghai had better waterways than Guangdong, so soon became the main silk export centre immediately after the War.[3] The region's raw silk exports rose from 5,146 to 46,655 piculs, while Guangdong's exports dropped from 5,430 to 3,662 piculs from 1845 to 1853.[4]

Through the century, the demand for Chinese silk further intensified, and the price soared, especially after French and Italian production suffered from silkworm disease in the 1850s.[5] The cocoon crop in France suddenly dropped from 19.8 to 7.7 million kilograms between 1855 and 1856 and then declined again to 5.5 million kilograms in 1865.[6] While raw silk production in France and Italy drastically decreased from 2,100 to 600 tons from 1853 to 1855, there was a stark decrease from 1,607 to 826 tons in Italy from 1863 to 1865.[7] However, global demand was increasing, as Europe and the United States became industrial powers in the nineteenth century, their purchasing power increased, and so did their demand for silk.[8] This intensified the demand for Chinese raw silk, driving the price up, reaching 340 taels (1 tael equivalent to $1.38 Spanish dollars) per picul (1 picul equivalent to 133.3 lbs) in Shanghai in 1859.[9] At the same time, production in the burgeoning Shanghai region also crashed during the Taiping rebellion (1851–1864), which was centred near the northern silk area of Jiangnan. As a result of the rebellion, the mulberry trees used to feed the silkworms and the silk looms were largely destroyed.[10] Consequently, production was severely diminished, and the price of silk continued to rise, reaching 500 taels per picul in 1866.[11] It was not until 1879 that Shanghai's silk exports recovered to the levels of the late 1850s.[12]

4.2.1 New Silk Production Hub in the Pearl River Delta

Growing demand and production issues elsewhere in China greatly benefitted the silk industry in the Pearl River Delta. The high profit of silk production attracted merchant attention in the Delta, where silk production dates back to as early as the Han dynasty (209–202 BC).[13] The climate and environmental conditions required to grow mulberry trees and rear silkworms were excellent in the delta. Mulberry leaves could grow quickly, giving eight yields a year, which provided enough food to feed the silkworms.[14] Silkworm rearing took 16 to 18 days only, and the region could produce triple the cocoon output compared to Jiangnan.[15] The great climate provided good conditions to establish a new major silk production hub in the Delta, focused on Shunde, in the late 1860s.[16] This hub would have excellent waterways and be located on Hong Kong's doorstep. Until the mid-nineteenth century, the economy of the delta was quite diversified in that no single crop dominated, with the exception of China's staple crop, rice. However, the profit from growing mulberry trees was approximately three to ten times higher than that of rice, so rice fields were transformed to mulberry cultivation.[17] Monocrop cultivation of mulberry trees began to take place in the 1860s, and land used for mulberry trees rose from 8,500 to 189,000 mou (1 mou equals 0.667 hectare) through the period of 1844 to 1867.[18] This large source of mulberry leaves was key to massive cocoon production, which formed the basis for the region's vibrant silk industry, which saw raw silk exports increase from 2,969 to 9,259 piculs from the early 1840s to 1867.

During this period, Chinese silk exports were basically under the control of Britain, which held the exclusive privilege to navigate the Chinese coast and inland waters after the First and Second Opium Wars (1839–1842 and 1856–1860). This allowed the British to go deep into China, to inland silk producing areas, and trade in Chinese raw silk heading for Europe. The silk was first transported to London via Hong Kong and then distributed to the silk mills located in Britain, France, and Italy from the beginning of the 1840s.[19] This pattern began to change at the turn of the 1860 and

1870s. With the opening of a direct service between the United States and Asia by the Pacific Mail Steamship Co in 1867, the opening of the Suez Canal in 1869, and the completion of the Far Eastern section of the submarine cable in 1871, transportation and communication around the world was greatly enhanced, facilitating the direct import of raw silk into Europe and the States from China.[20] All these improvements combined to induce an expansion of Chinese raw silk exports to the West, impelling major changes in China's economy and silk industry and further incorporating them into the world system.

China became the raw silk supplier to the world, supplying silk mills in Europe and the United States from the 1870s.[21] The production of cocoons and raw silk gradually recovered in Europe over that decade, with Italy's raw silk production expanding from 2,366 to 3,200 tons from 1873 to 1883 to within 90 percent of the previous peak, but the recovery of France's raw silk industry had not yet come.[22] In the meantime, the consumption of silk shifted from luxury commodities to daily use commodities, such as pyjamas. By this time, France had a high demand for raw silk; however, its domestic production could only supply a small portion of that demand. In 1874, France consumed one-third of the total world consumption of raw silk,[23] and by 1880, France imported half of its demand from China.[24] Similarly, there was a rise in demand for silk commodities in the United States, which could not depend on domestic supply either, so had to import the shortfall. Thereafter, the country's raw silk imports from China increased tenfold in the ten years between 1869 (102,000 lbs) and 1879.[25] In 1860, the proportion of different commodities exported from China to the United States was 68.2% (tea) and 3.6% (raw silk), but silk (35%) overtook tea (34.7%) as the leading export commodity by 1901, and that trend continued until 1911, when silk was 39.7% and tea was 8.4%.[26]

China's raw silk exports were 45.6, 39.8 and 31% of world raw silk exports for the periods of 1870–1874, 1895–1899 and 1910–1914, respectively.[27] Its position as the largest raw silk supplier was not surpassed until 1905–1909 by Japan.[28] From 1921 to 1929, during the Great Depression (beginning in the United States in the late 1920s and spreading to Europe), an average of 58.8 and 40.8% of Chinese raw silk was exported to the United States and Europe per year, respectively.[29] China's silk exports were principally raw silk, which was approximately 76% of its total silk exports between 1868 and 1912.[30] In this respect, a similar figure shows that 80% of the Chinese silk export value came from raw silk from 1882 to 1931.[31] In 1874, the value of 68,400 piculs amounted to 1,946 Haikwan taels (1 Haikwan tael equivalent to $0.79 US dollars), rising to 83,200 piculs and 2,728 Haikwan taels in 1894. This dramatic increase in value was eight times that in the 1840s.[32] Raw silk exports from Guangdong accounted for only 8% of total Chinese silk exports (in picul) in 1859,[33] which soon jumped to 31.6% in 1870 and peaked at 38.9% in 1895 (Table 4.2). Clearly, China's economy was highly dependent on raw silk exports.

Despite China's raw silk being well received in the world market, the variation in quality and strength produced by the traditional hand-reeling production method hampered manufacturing capacity and depressed the price, as the nonstandardized quality and strength was not suitable for the mass production machinery used in the West.[34] Responding to foreign tastes and aiming to maintain competition in overseas

Table 4.2 Percentage of Guangdong silk exports of total China silk export, 1870–1920

	China raw silk export (picul)	Guangdong raw silk export (%)
1870	49,160	15,535 (31.6)
1885	57,984	21,203 (36.6)
1895	110,621	42,989 (38.9)
1905	105,919	32,000 (30.2)
1910	139,226	44,638 (32)
1915	143,097	33,000 (23)
1920	104,315	34,000 (32.6)

Source Li, 1981: 71–6; Lau, 2006: 66, 139; Wong, 2017:180, 187–90

markets, Guangdong and Shanghai were the first two places in China to industrialize silk production through the introduction of steam-reeling machinery in the 1860s and the 1870s, respectively.[35] By 1886, Shunde in the Delta had 42 silk factories, which expanded to 142 by 1911.[36] Following such intensification of the industry in the second half of the century, the national cultivation of mulberry trees specialized in the delta, as seen in the production of mulberry leaves and cocoons and the demand for cultivated land (Table 4.3). Half of 'the cultivated land in Shunde came to be used for mulberry tree plantations,[37] which was key to cocoon production, and the delta came to contribute half of Guangdong's cocoon production.[38] A European travel writer of the time noted widespread silk production in the delta,

> In this delta country, there are at least 1,000 square miles that are devoted almost entirely to the growth of mulberries. One can travel for a day on a passage boat through the region and see nothing but mulberry fields...[39]

Table 4.3 Guangdong silk industry production and silk exports, 1839–1934

Year	Mulberry cultivation (mou)	Mulberry leaf production (picul)	Cocoon production (picul)	Raw silk export (picul)
1839–1844	8,500	212,000	2,970	416
1850–1853	60,000 (706%)	1,515,000 (715%)	21,200 (714%)	2,969 (714%)
1860	114,000 (190%)	2,842,000 (188%)	39,800 (188%)	5,571 (188%)
1867	189,000 (186%)	4,724,000 (166%)	66,100 (166%)	9,259 (166%)
1895–1899	596,000 (315%)	14,900,000 (315%)	209,000 (316%)	29,216 (316%)
1910–1914	811,000 (136%)	20,310,000 (136%)	284,000 (136%)	39,800 (136%)
1925–1929	1,040,000 (128%)	26,000,000 (128%)	364,000 (128%)	51,000 (128%)
1930–1934	699,000 (−67%)	17,475,000 (−67%)	245,000 (−67%)	34,250 (−67%)

Source So, 1986: 80.
Note The percentage in the brackets is the percentage change compared to the previous year or period

In the case of silk, China's integration into the world economy drove local industrialization. Much of the silk exported from China to the West was raw, which made it the top world raw silk supplier for Western factories of woven silk commodities from 1870 to 1905, which came to rely heavily on the new world silk market. Instead of following a dependency perspective that industries in peripheral areas are destroyed when incorporated into the capitalist world system, Alvin So describes the industrialization of China's silk production as 'peripheral industrialization' to differentiate the process from industrialization in core countries. Peripheral industrialization characterizes the influence of the world market on China's silk industry, while industrializing, China could only respond to core demand and so could not control its own development.[40] Nevertheless, while China kept its silk industry, it was impossible for the country to avoid demand fluctuations in the world silk market due to market saturation or demand shrinkage, causing declines in the raw silk price.[41] For instance, a fall in price occurred in 1877 because of overstocking in Europe.[42] More specifically, the price in Shanghai suddenly dropped from 500 to 285 Haikwan taels between 1873 and 1875, and the price decreased 27% from 1871 to 1881.[43] The result was clearly a vicious cycle; the price dropped from US$1,500 to US$1,000 per picul in the early 1920s to the end of the decade, the beginning of the Great Depression.[44]

4.2.2 Silk, Night Soil and Public Toilet

Such large exports reflect the extensive cultivation of mulberry trees, which increased the demand for night soil, turning Hong Kong's public toilet infrastructure into night soil collection points by the late 1860s. Whereas bodily waste in public was considered to be dirt and a nuisance to the urban environment, the night soil sitting in public toilets was valued as fertilizer. This highlights the supply chain within the world system. Hong Kong night soil was used to fertilize Shunde's mulberry trees. Then, Shunde raw silk was exported to Europe and the United States via Hong Kong, and woven Western silk commodities were exported around the world, including back to China.[45] This section does not intend to detail the entire Chinese silk industry; instead, the aim is to briefly understand the influence that the world silk market had in driving the expansive cultivation of mulberry trees and industrial development in southern China, boosting demand for night soil. The historical circumstances of the rise of a favorable world silk market set the stage for establishing an export-oriented silk production hub in the delta; only with such a market for silk was the citywide provision of public toilets possible in Hong Kong from late 1860 to 1930. In tandem, the fluctuations in night soil demand, caused by the silk industry's own instabilities, complicated the sustainability of toilet services.

As a vast agrarian country, soil fertility has long been a major concern in China.[46] Compared to livestock dung, human excrement contains much more nitrogen and phosphorus and has been treated as a superior fertilizer by farmers to produce high-quality crops and increase yield.[47] For these reasons, the use of human excrement in cultivation goes back to as early as the Yuan dynasty in 1239–1368.[48] The increased quality and quantity of plant growth was especially critical for mulberry trees, as high-quality leaves fed to silkworms would produce high-quality silk; furthermore, the quantity of leaves was the primary bottleneck for silk production. Moreover, the amount of fertilizer applied to mulberry fields was much higher than that applied to other crops, such as cotton, rice or wheat.[49] As such, a large quantity of city night soil, which had a higher quality, was required in Shunde. These combined factors led to a high demand for Hong Kong night soil from Delta's mulberry tree growers.

The cross-border night soil business between Hong Kong and the Delta was then formed, and the sale of night soil became a lucrative business from the late 1860s to the early twentieth century. During this period, while Hong Kong was a British colony, the border between it and Shunde was relatively open before 1949, after which China fell under the control of the Communist Party and the border was progressively strengthened.[50] Such an open border supported a high level of movement of goods and people. At the time, it was quite common for mainland Chinese merchants to travel as far as 70 miles to purchase quality night soil to resell to farmers in mainland China.[51] At a distance of approximately 65 miles, Hong Kong was near enough to Shunde.[52] Urban night soil was highly prized by Shunde farmers, making the colony's night soil highly profitable. For example, in 1882, the sale price for night soil in China was HK$0.15 to 0.20 per picul,[53] and the price increased to HK$0.70 by 1898, as mentioned in Chapter One. The night soil in government-owned and privately owned toilets was the respective property of either the contractors or toilet operators; therefore, the contractors had to tender the night soil deposited in government toilets, and the tender price was HK$0.23 to $0.28 between 1898 and 1899.[54]

The widespread silk production in China inevitably drove demand for night soil, but this was ultimately driven by the wider context of the world silk market of European and North American demand. The attractiveness of night soil profits led Chinese merchants and the government to become actively involved in the night soil market, sprouting many supporting businesses in the capitalist turn of sanitation. Driven by market forces, toilets were commodified as night soil collection points, which supplied a critical boost to the night soil industry while also increasing revenue to the government and business while solving the colony's public defecation problem. This hints that night soil revenue was an economic incentive to provide sanitation services, especially in the form of commercial public toilets (both government and privately owned).

4.3 Involvement of Government in Night Soil Business

High night soil profits not only increased business enthusiasm to collect it and encouraged people into the toilet market but also created a strong incentive for the government to transform government toilets into night soil collection points by introducing the night soil tender system. In the first two years (1867–1868) of the government public toilet program, an annual payment was paid by the government to night soil contractors for night soil removal. For example, HK$960 was charged in 1868.[55] As night soil became valuable in 1869, Au Cheung Li, the former night soil contractor for government public toilets in 1867, joined with Lo Chuk Shang, a pork butcher, and successfully tendered a bid of HK$240 for the night soil deposited in government public toilets and buildings.[56] The government went from paying for removal to selling the opportunity to remove the night soil. Well aware of the value of night soil in Shunde, the contractors were happy to purchase the night soil from the government instead of charging a removal fee. These numbers suggest that the profit of selling night soil in China was higher than HK$1,200 (the total of HK$240 and HK$960). At that time, there was no competition from other bidders; therefore, Au and Lo successfully purchased night soil at a low price.

4.3.1 Night Soil Tendering System and Night Soil Revenue

The value of night soil and a very limited colony budget pushed the government to provide toilet services on a profitable basis through the tendering of night soil. The government soon sold the night soil from its toilets in public areas and government buildings as different night soil contracts, institutionalizing night soil collection as a business model. Such a move created the night soil contractor business, a critical player in a functioning public toilet market. Under the tender system, collection rights were granted to the highest bidder, who had to pay the government a yearly fee for the right to collect the night soil, as well as clear dirt and dust from public dustbins.[57] This model was arranged with the expectation that tendering would sustain free night soil removal and subsidize toilet services for users, which would operate on a quasi-commercial basis while contributing to urban hygiene. This model also generated much-needed revenue for the government to meet any expenses (e.g., the cost of providing oil lamps and brooms) related to maintaining toilet facilities. The successful bidders had to pay the government in advance on the first day of each month, or every six months, and were also heavily bonded, with two guarantors given by Chinese elites such as compradors, shopkeepers, traders, PLK or TWH directors. Furthermore, there was a bond, for example, of HK$4,000 for a contract of HK$9,800 in 1885.[58]

In Hong Kong, government toilets therefore became commercialized and were therefore blended with capitalist concerns through the institutionalization of the night soil market. In China, however, the institutional sale of night soil was centrally managed as early as the late Ming dynasty.[59] However, the more capitalist tendering system used in the colony originated in the West. To finance night soil removal and public toilet services, human excrement was often put to public auctions in Britain, France and the United States by the governments in the nineteenth century.[60] The practice was also replicated in Western colonies and foreign settlements. Due to the great demand for night soil as fertilizer, when mulberry and cotton became cash crops in the late Qing dynasty (1636–1912), the night soil collection monopolies always tended to be a number of local businesses in foreign settlements located in China.[61]

Similarly, the Hong Kong colonial government came to be involved as an economic actor in the night soil business. Perhaps the most obvious way it was involved in this business was in its role as the owner of the night soil that was to be collected from government public toilets and buildings. The development of the market was thus accelerated and institutionalized by the government, and it was here that night soil speculation developed. Along with the burgeoning silk industry and increasing demand for night soil in Shunde, market speculation increased demand and prices in this small colony. Chinese merchants were happy to join the night soil business, as the resource monopoly system delivered "the possibility of great wealth" to contractors. There are two major indicators of great wealth being made, the first of which was vibrant bids. In view of the great profit of night soil, night soil tenders were very competitive, and a total of twenty-nine tenders were collected in 1870.[62] Night soil price inflation is reflected in the wide bids of contractors, which ranged from HK$400 to HK$1,656. The successful bid for the year 1872 was HK$2,750.[63] One bidder at the time claimed he would even bid HK$4,000 if the government allowed him to pay the charges at the year end, instead of half-yearly in advance, so that he could collect night soil debts from Chinese farmers after harvest periods.

Although many of the contractors came from rather humble origins, they still frequently had connections with Chinese elites. When Chan Kam tendered for the night soil monopoly in 1898,[64] his guarantors were Tong Wan Chiu, comprador to Measieurs Sander Wieler, the directors of PLK (1894/1895) and TWH (1895/1896),[65] and Ku Fai Shan, managing partner of Po Lung Firm (a dealer in Chinese goods for the American market); more details about the latter will be provided in later sections. Chan Pui's guarantors were Fung Wah Chuen and Tang Pak Shan in 1889.[66] Fung was a PLK director and chairman (1884/1885, 1894/1895, 1899/1900 and 1903/1904), TWH director and chairman (1892/1893, 1897/1898 and 1901/1902), and the first chairman of the Chinese Chamber of Commerce in the early 1900s; he was also a JP from 1902 to 1907.[67] Tang Pak Shan was a trader and son of Tang Luk[68]; see Chap. 2 for the latter's background. Later, Chan Pui rented a toilet at 29 First Street from Tang.[69] Without socioeconomic connections, it was impossible for these contractors to successfully win a tender, which is why a limited number of contractors such as Chan Pui and Kwong Kam Tong were repeatedly granted the tenders and enjoyed the profits.[70]

The second major indicator for great wealth is the scale of the business. Ho A Chak, the successful bidder in 1872 mentioned above, operated 22 conservancy boats to transport the night soil up the delta. Chan Pui, who started as a scavenging contractor responsible for emptying rubbish bins at the Slaughter House in Kennedy Town in 1884, later extended his waste collecting business to night soil in 1889 and then surface scavenging in 1893.[71] He came to run a large night soil operation, employing 48 boatmen, 45 nightmen, 13 foremen and watchmen, and nine public toilet attendants.[72] This kind of organizational size indicates that the night soil business sector was not small. After accumulating wealth over a decade, in the mid-1890s, Chan significantly entered the public toilet market, renting and owning a number of toilets, and purchasing land in Wanchai as well, which shall be covered more later. A contemporary account sheds light on the wealth available, Catherine Joyce Symons, a former headmistress at Diocesan Girls' School in the 1980s, recalled her memories as a student at the school in the 1930s: "the father of one of my school friends had successfully tendered for the job of collecting all the night-soil on Hong Kong Island and became very rich indeed".[73] The evidence demonstrates that night soil collection was a highly profitable business venture.

Significant night soil revenue was collected by both private contractors and the government. The night soil business in Hong Kong was particularly vibrant in the period between the 1880s and early 1900s (Fig. 4.2), and it was during this period that night soil was significant enough to government revenue to be reported separately. Night soil revenue between 1869 and 1886 was not recorded, as it was too small, a mere HK$240. However, from 1887 to 1903, the government separately reported night soil revenue under the item "Night Soil Contracts".[74] During this period, night soil revenue dramatically increased to HK$67,920 in 1902. The Night Soil Contracts entry initially only included revenue from government buildings, but after the 1880s, it came to include profits from private houses in areas outside Victoria City and animal manure from public markets.[75] Night soil revenue was then recategorized as "Conservancy Contracts" from 1904 until 1930.[76] In 1902, night soil contracts accounted for approximately 1.39 percent of the total yearly budget, and there was an average of 1 percent or more of yearly revenue of the total budget until the early twentieth century. The overall farming system of tendered monopolies, including night soil collection and exporting opium, provided up to 10 to 25 percent of annual revenue from the 1840s to the 1870s, as shown in Chap. 2. Clearly, government public toilets were a financial success in that the toilet service was not only financially sustainable but also provided much-needed revenue.

These numbers show only a small proportion of Hong Kong's total night soil industry and the revenues that it generated, as they do not include the private contractors and operators who came to dominate that industry. The government's revenue (generated from government public toilets and household night soil buckets) was double that of the private public toilet market.[77] While the government did generate an income from its public toilets, it's stated goal, as shown in Chap. 3, was to stem the outbreak of deadly disease. In practice, this meant to address the worst ongoing sanitation issues in the Chinese quarter, contemporary Sheung Wan, Saiyingpun and Kennedy Town, which was politically deemed to be a disease breeding ground. The quarter also happened to be the location of tenements for lower-class Chinese that lacked domestic toilets. Thus, the locations of the first five toilets were situated at Saiyingpun Market, Shektongtsui Market, Western Market in Sheung Wan, and Cattle Depot and Slaughter House in Kennedy Town.[78] However, development beyond these initial five toilets was slow, and there were no more built until the mid-1880s, and then only two more added, for a total of seven in 1885.[79] The new locations were Sokonpo (Causeway Bay) and Caine Road (Central Mid-levels).[80] In 1891, a further four were built for a total of eleven, but then this remained the status quo until the end of the century.[81] In contrast, the private toilet market boomed.

The value of night soil for business was much greater than for the government; as mentioned, 75% of toilet seats were privately owned at the peak of the industry. The huge night soil takings of private enterprises caught the government's attention, which

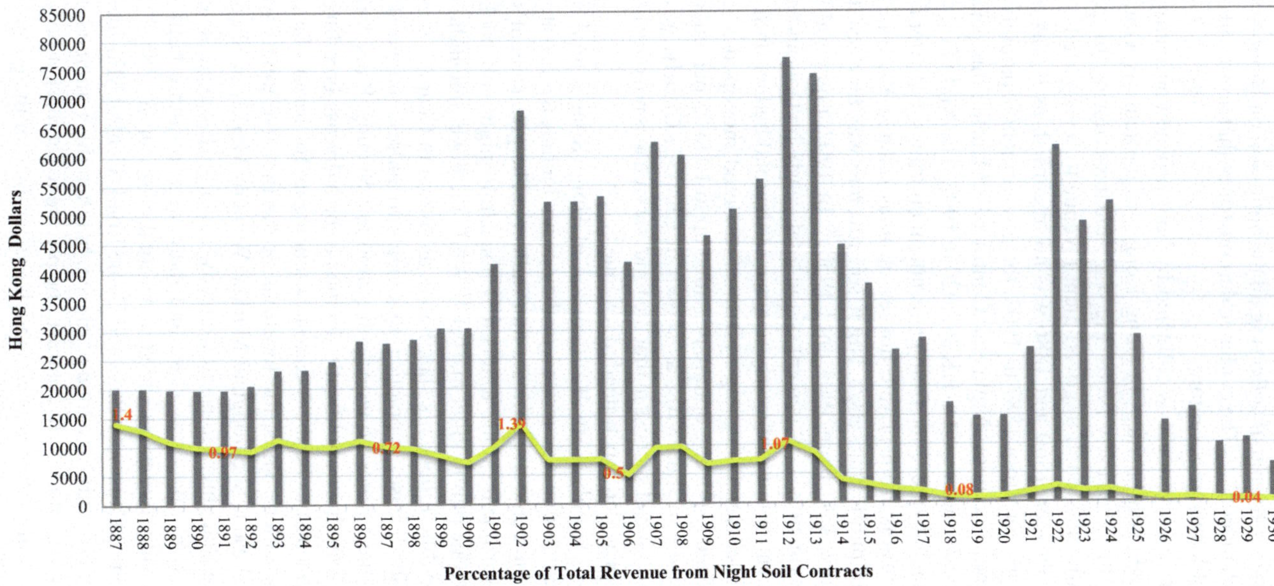

Fig. 4.2 Government Night Soil Revenue, 1887–1930 (HK$). *Source* The author compiled the percentages from the following documents: Night Soil Contract, *BB*, 1887–1903; Conservancy Contract, *BB*, 1904–1930; Comparative Yearly State of the Revenue, *BB*, 1887–1930

led to the government contesting ownership of the night soil profits. In an attempt to monopolize the colony's night soil markets and raise revenue, the government proposed putting c privately owned toilets under its control. At the turn of the century, it was estimated that such a plan would increase government night soil revenue by 50%, from HK$30,384 to HK$46,100, combined with revenue from government toilets and household night soil buckets.[82] Although the estimation was attractive and the Sanitary Board highly recommended that the government should take over privately run public toilets, the plan was turned down. The crucial point was that these toilets were mostly situated in valuable locations, which made their resumption cost high, as the loss of night soil profit to the private owners would be very large. More importantly, the proposed arrangement would have deprived business owners of considerable revenue from the sale of night soil. The resumption would surely stir resentment among them, who either way was accustomed to opposing urban public health measures that conflicted with their interests, as shown in Chap. 3. To a certain extent, collaboration with business in public toilets limited the ability of the government to intervene in the provision and exercise any public health measures. The government had to trade some of its authority, but this did not mean that it was no longer autonomous. It is important not to neglect that the government still had several means to influence toilet operation, for example, legal and supervisory powers (more will be discussed in Chap. 5).

The government played a crucial role in developing a market economy of toilets. The government's direct involvement in the night soil business—instituting the night soil tender—is crucial to understand how it facilitated the capitalist turn of public toilets as night soil collection points and understand the subsequent urban governance of toilet services that operated between the government and Chinese business. The important role of the government in the commercialization of public toilets must be noted in two aspects. First is its involvement as both an economic and political actor in "public toilet economies". In this regard, by instituting the night soil monopoly and tendering system of its own collected night soil, the government moved the night soil business from being purely private to partially in public. Tendering led to an institutional change in the prevailing public health logic. Marketization had the paradoxical effect of promoting night soil price inflation while dramatically transforming public toilets from being purely public health facilities to night soil collection points. Second, the attractiveness of the night soil profits led the government to become actively involved in the night soil business and support Chinese businesses (night soil contractors, toilet operators and toilet landowners) in operating privately owned toilets for night soil profit by establishing wharves that facilitated the business.[83] To fulfil both moral (toilet cleanliness) and economic (maintain the manurial value of night soil, collect toilet entrance fees and rental returns) aims, the government introduced an inspectorate system to supervise night soil removal and toilet daily operation (see details in Chap. 5). Enabled by a capitalist economy, the night soil profits were significant for enabling commercial toilet provision (both government and private owned). However, this had an apparent effect on their character, so that the toilets were not merely a moral space operated in the public interest but rather were operated on a quasi-commercial basis.

In purchasing night soil to fertilize their mulberry trees in nearby Guangdong, the Chinese business established the demand for Hong Kong's night soil and provided the source of wealth that sustained public toilets. The high value of night soil allowed the colonial government to leave the problem of providing and managing public toilets in the hands of business. The government not only sold the rights to collect the night soil deposited in government toilets to night soil contractors but also protected the rights of private owners of night soil in privately owned toilets. This market-oriented public toilet approach of the government helped to boost the market forces that supported the provision of quasi-commercial public toilets. Up until the early twentieth century, when night soil demand continued to rise, commercial toilets (both government-owned and privately owned) were the dominant sanitation method in Hong Kong.[84] It was very clear that the high value at night could serve as a mechanism to mediate the interests between the government and business in terms of public toilet provision.

4.3.2 Cross-Border Night Soil Business Operation

The cross-border night soil business operated in the following closely linked ways: night soil contractors recruited coolies (on a piece rate basis) to remove the night soil from both government-owned and privately owned public toilets. The number of coolies engaged in the night soil business was probably approximately 500 in the early 1880s.[85] Their income depended on the number of piculs of night soil they removed, which was HK$0.05 to HK$0.10 per picul in 1899.[86] These coolies were self-employed, not employees of the contractors or of the government, and therefore were not under the control of the government. After the outbreak of the plague in 1894, the coolie licensing system was introduced, which meant that contractors could only employ licenced coolies to remove night soil.[87] Under the system, coolies were licenced annually by the Sanitary Board, and they were required to wear a badge and only use a specific bucket design approved by the Board. Furthermore, they had to move night soil between 1 A.M. However, the use of hardwood buckets with closely fitting lids, as ordered by the Board, triggered a strike by the coolies in 1896 when the licensing system was more effectively enforced.[88] To better manage the coolies, they were allowed to elect yearly a committee of representatives of no more than 12 from among them. That committee then assisted the Board in exercising strict supervision over the licenced coolies.

Starting from 1 A.M. daily, night soil coolies collected night soil from toilets, they then collected the night soil into their larger buckets, next at between 2:30 A.M. and 7 A.M. In summer, they took the night soil to the conservancy boats, and the material was then transported to an anchorage.[89] By the early twentieth century, the boats had to be registered annually with the Sanitary Board.[90] To facilitate night soil removal, as noted, in 1867, the government built ten wharves, which were scattered along the foreshore of Hong Kong Island covering the middle to western part of Causeway Bay, Central and Saiyingpun. The wharves may have originally been established to dump the night soil into the water before the night soil business began, similar to how rubbish was thrown on the beach in westernmost Hong Kong at the time.[91] Different wharves catered to boats with different carrying capacities in picul weight, for example the wharves in Jardine Bazaar (today Causeway Bay) and Ship Street in Wanchai catered for boats with capacities of 100 and 600 piculs, respectively.[92] The contractors had to provide boats suitable in number and carrying capacity, ranging from 100 to 600 piculs, while the crew of each boat depended on its size, ranging from three to eight men.[93]

The night soil was exported by conservancy boats flying a naval flag decided by the Sanitary Board. The boats delivered the night soil to Stonecutters Island in western Hong Kong. The night soil contractors were only allowed to resell the night soil from their conservancy boats after the boats had reached the Island, and the purchase must be done before 1 P.M.[94] The night soil had to be loaded onto the larger vessels no later than 2 P.M.[95] The night soil would then be gathered on the island daily and then transported to Shunde on a regular basis two to three times a week. Night soil destined for Shunde was delivered to nearby Wong Lin through the Bocca Tigris channel, which was a night soil depot that was easily accessible to the Shunde waterways where the night soil awaited distribution around the silk-producing areas (Fig. 4.3).

In the early 1880s, 57,738 piculs of night soil (from government-owned and privately owned public toilets and dwellings) were collected per year.[96] By the end of the century, the amount yield from toilets per annum had reached 184,000 piculs, solely from public toilets.[97] Rapid urbanization and dramatic population growth at the time, as noted in previous chapters, declined the amount of agricultural land in Hong Kong, so the local night soil demand declined accordingly, making sanitation an

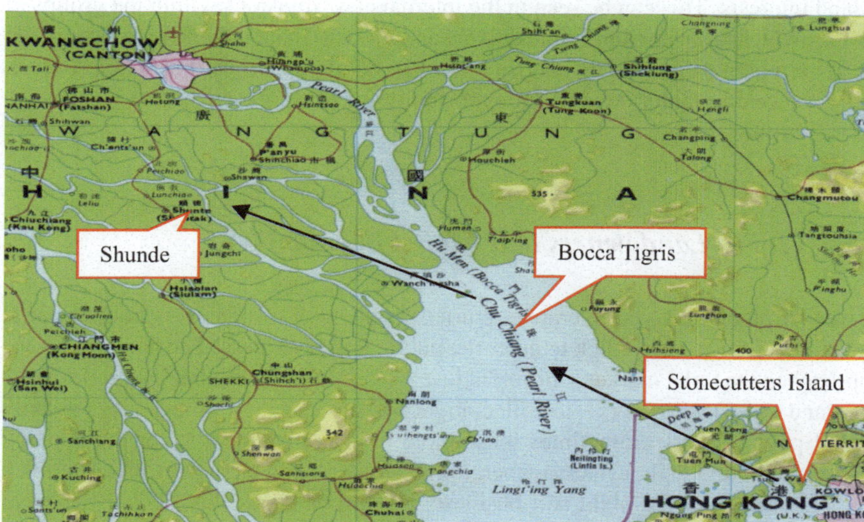

Fig. 4.3 Cross-border night soil transportation route

urgent issue that needs to be addressed, especially among lower-class Chinese people who were living in tenement houses without toilets. The high demand for night soil in Shunde dovetailed with the large quantity of surplus night soil being produced in rapidly growing Hong Kong. The total civil population reached 241,762 (233,280 Chinese) in 1897, and the high urban density (noted in Chap. 3) offered a huge, collectable supply.[98] Indeed, there are many studies on the matter of turning public toilets into night soil collection points, regulating urban space, and saving the public finances of colonies in Asia.[99] The public toilets of the time were a valuable urban property that existed in a symbiotic relationship with the countryside, whose farmers purchased their contents to use as night soil fertilizer. As Xue notes, the night soil business "served as a sewage system for the urban area", as traders removed the waste for their own profit while maintaining public health and a clean neighbourhood,[100] further increasing property values for landowners. This is seen in the nineteenth century profit-driven toilet provision of Hong Kong, underpinned by the collection of city night soil. Toilet services correlated closely with the wider context of the world silk industry and silk production in the Pearl River Delta.

4.4 Marketing Moral Space: The Profit of Urban Land

The commercialization of public toilets was shaped not only by night soil profits but also by those of land. In the new economic reality, centred on land investment, the growing importance of land revenue for government and business resulted in the two types of public toilets, government-owned and privately owned, becoming entangled in land interests. This can be seen in the internal class divisions within the groups of government, Europeans and Chinese over sanitation in Chap. 3. Land profits attracted the government to auction the lands rather than taking up a role of service provider, being a service enabler creating an opportunity for homemade Chinese business to enter the toilet market.

4.4.1 Toilet-Landowners and "Toilet Economies"

Driven by potentially very lucrative returns, people with sufficient economic capital and land holdings were quick to enter the public toilet business. The business sector approached the toilet market at different levels—as night soil contractors, toilet operators and toilet landowners—to collect night soil or lease their property as privately owned public toilets. Sometimes these three roles were transitory or overlapping for a single individual business owner. For example, being a contractor was a quick way to understand the night soil business, which could possibly deliver the great wealth offered by the night soil monopolies. After accumulating enough wealth, some contractors would then enter the public toilet market proper by either renting or purchasing a privately owned public toilet property to directly collect the night soil and maximize their returns. Being a contractor was a steppingstone to becoming a toilet operator or even a toilet landowner. In reality, however, the transitions were more complex, as some held two to three positions (such as Chan Pui) at the same time.

Like other government night soil contractors such as Tso Po To (who was a contractor in 1870 and then had his own toilet by 1882),[101] Chan Pui was also happy to work in the toilet market for the lucrative investment opportunity. Chan was first a scavenging contractor at Slaughter House in Kennedy Town in 1884 and later extended his waste collecting business to night soil in 1889 and then ground surface scavenging (collecting refuse, animal manure and night soil from the villages in Kowloon Peninsular) in 1893.[102] After building a small fortune, he entered the toilet market in the early 1890s, purchasing the facility at 14 Mercer Street in Sheung Wan, and renting three more at 2 Gough Street in Sheung Wan, 256 Queens Road West and 3 Sam To Lane in Saiyingpun.[103] As an operator and landowner of privately owned toilets, which were directly targeted towards collecting night soil, it was not an exaggeration for people to call him the "Night Soil Lord". As the owner or rentier of four toilets, Chan Pui's wealth definitely attracted attention; for example, he was repeatedly extorted by a European Sanitary Inspector for over a hundred dollars from 1904 to 1906.[104] Furthermore, Chan was involved in a court case of alleged bribery of a civil servant; fortunately, he was pronounced innocent, while the inspector was charged with accepting bribes.

Under land-centered capitalism, land resources were the crucial resource for the involvement of wealthy Chinese in the toilet market. As the owners of land, it was these people who provided the land for toilet facilities, so they played a critical role in defining who could have access to public toilets by deciding the location of such facilities. Furthermore, in the next chapter, we will see that they strategically sustained their toilets through the establishment of "spheres of influence" that contained the miasma and other nuisances (e.g., foul smell) of such facilities. In doing so, landowners freed the government from needing to negotiate facility locations with other powerful landowners, who would often oppose the establishment of a government public toilet. Through their actions, these landowners transcended the colonizer-colonized and public–private spheres. They served a public function by helping to regulate lower-class Chinese people's use of urban space. This study therefore focuses on toilet landowners, rather than contractors or operators, as the scarcity of land made both the toilet operators and the government incapable of being independent of this landed class.

The government-business collaboration relationship was a very strong sense of common self-interest in urban space, so urban order was always restructured by the racial and class politics of that collaboration. In practice, the drive to provide toilet services for the lower-class Chinese also involved both political and economic concerns. This indicates the complexity of colonial spatial relations in two ways. First, the landowners' position of being Chinese meant that they were standing at the crossroads of race and class, helping the government solve the problem of lower-class Chinese defecating in public places. Second, they controlled much land, which allowed them to maintain a negotiated relationship with the government over toilet provision. As land resources were concentrated in the hands of a small group of Chinese landowners, their use of collective land power in constraining and facilitating public toilets was significantly improved. This helped to maintain the sustainability of privately owned toilets through a web of social networks (see Chap. 5 for details) but also made toilet provision more political, as the government had to depend on them for toilet services. As such reliance strengthened the landowners' bargaining power over the government, the public health logic and moral geography of the colony was reformed.

Chinese landowners did not just run public toilets for profit, and there were many other advantages. While the high profit meant that some landowners were eager to take up the public role of public toilet providers, equally worth noting is that the emergence of capitalist development created the conditions for landowner self-interest, inducing them to act as active social agents in providing toilets to their fellow countrymen. The urgent need to regulate how lower-class Chinese used urban space, with the growing pressure posed by the potential threat of their bodily waste, was required not only by the government to protect European and economic prosperity but also by Chinese landowners to maintain clean neighbourhoods with high property values. Through the early period, lower-class Chinese were identified by the colonial government and Chinese elites as "unhygienic bodies" that caused disease and were a sanitary threat, which would depreciate property values. For Chinese business elites, the issue was particularly acute, as their property investments were mostly in the same neighbourhoods as the homes of lower-class Chinese. Furthermore, during the Hennessy administration, these landowners bought land and built many shops and tenements, incentivizing them to offer public toilets to contain bodily waste. Furthermore, providing toilets was also important to reducing the pressure to construct domestic toilets in tenement housing buildings, which would maximize rentable space. A class division is reflected in the provision of privately owned toilets, which not only set elite and lower-class Chinese physically a part (elites distinguished themselves through the use of home night soil buckets and better public toilets) but also conceptually a part in terms of bodily habits and the eligibility of using both domestic and public toilets.

By the mid-nineteenth century, as mentioned in Chap. 2, the Chinese were increasing their landholdings, as shown in the government rate books, toilet landowners' wills, and their estates, they possessed huge land holdings. This was conducive to landowners' participation in toilet provision. The author compiled the land records in rate books and computed the pieces of land based on the names of eight main toilet landowners (Choy Chan, Ip Ching Chuen, Kwok Acheong, Ng Ping Sam, Pow Ping Kwan, Tang Luk, Tso Wing Yung, and Tsui Cheong Lung) and their family members from rate books between 1877 and 1895.[105] The numbers of land properties for 1877, 1880, 1888, and 1895 were 385, 338, 478 and 434, respectively. Furthermore, it has already been discussed that Chinese elites who had heavily invested in land became the top taxpayers in 1876 and 1881. Undoubtedly, some of them were landowners of private toilets. In 1876, eight Chinese were among the top twenty taxpayers, of which five were involved in the toilet market.[106] The highest taxpayer among these landowners was Kwok Acheong (HK$6,906, ranked

No. 3), followed by Cheng Sing Yeung (HK$5,730, No. 9), Choy Chan (HK$2,988, No. 13), Tso Wing Yung (HK$2,585, No. 15) and Ng Sang (HK$2,572, No. 16). Five years later, there were seventeen Chinese in the top twenty taxpayers, of which six were toilet landowners.[107] The list was Ng Sang (HK$10,240, No. 2), Kwok's sons Kwok Yin Kai (HK$5,748, No. 8) and Kwok Yin Shew (HK$4,700, No. 14), Tang Luk (HK$4,748, No. 14), Ip Ching Chuen (HK$4,156, No. 17) and Choy Chan (HK$4,048, No. 18). Two of them were present in the top twenty in both 1876 and 1881: Choy Chan and Ng Sang, the latter of which saw a dramatic increase in their payment, their contribution growing from HK$2,572, ranked sixteenth, to HK$10,240, ranked second.

The top taxpayer's estates were also huge, much of it held in property across Victoria City. For example, Tso Wing Yung left an estate of HK$118,000 in 1876, and there were many others, including Kwok Acheong (HK$445,000, 1880), Pang Wa (HK$5,000, 1883), Tang Luk (HK$208,699, 1887) and his son Tang Tung Shang (HK$300,750, 1894), Ip Ching Chuen (HK$208,100, 1889), Choy Chan (HK$1,021,384, 1904) and Pow Ping Kwan (HK$163,403, 1905).[108] Prominent among those was Choy Chan, as shown in Chap. 2. In the late 1890s, Choy entered a partnership with Lau Wai Chuen, who was compradored of the Hong Kong and Shanghai Bank, partnered of Tung Shang Wo (California and Australian Exporter's Firm) and JP in 1904, to purchase properties. Lau was also chairman of PLK (1887/1888) and TWH (1893/1894).[109] When a reclamation scheme was completed, Choy leased out fourteen shops along Connaught Road Central and Des Voeux Road Central to Tong Lai Chuen, who eventually became his executor. Tong was comprador to Shewan, Tomes & Co., JP and director of PLK (1898/1899; 1904/1905) and TWH (1894/1895).[110] These huge land resources allowed the landowners to lease the required properties as privately owned public toilets and sustain these facilities with "spheres of influence" (which will be discussed in Chap. 5) in the Chinese quarter when public health entangled land interests.

4.4.2 The Entanglement of Land Interests and Public Health

Chadwick knew well the great difficulties in achieving government public toilet provision in Hong Kong, where "the great cost of land does not give much opportunity for so doing".[111] Due to the high value of land, we have seen the government was reluctantly to construct sanitation infrastructure on Crown land. If infrastructure was provided, it was more often done to facilitate and enhance land sales than to actually improve sanitation. This can be seen in a dispatch sent by Governor H. Robinson (1859–1865) to the Permanent Under-Secretary of Government for the Colonies, F. Rogers Bart, in 1863. Robinson wrote, "sales of land render it necessary for the Government to undertake roads, streets, bridges, general drainage, public piers, and other works, without which the land either would not sell" and emphasized that "without such expenditure there would have been no surplus".[112] Perhaps the best way to explain this situation is that land-centered capitalism increased the importance of land revenue in political and economic structures and introduced an aspect of profit maximization to colonial rule. Under the high value of land and the government's laissez-faire attitude toward urban health governance, available land was often sold instead of being used for municipal purposes such as sanitation.[113] These profit concerns compelled the government to solve the sanitary problem by producing hygiene spaces under the terms of liberal economic orthodoxy, operating the public toilets on a quasi-commercial mode and putting the toilets in the hands of Chinese business.

Surprisingly, at least two years before the government introduced its first government public toilet in 1867, it attempted to encourage Chinese elites (for example Tepo) to offer toilet services for the Chinese community. During 1844–1861, the government set up the Tepo system, whereby the head male of each village or neighborhood helped to deal with local disputes, collect land rates, and manage burial grounds in certain districts.[114] As Lindblom notes, governments recognized that business requires encouragement to perform public functions in the form of incentives such as market or political benefits.[115] Guided by the hope of maintaining a minimal level of sanitation in the Chinese quarter at no expense to public funds and crown land use in the long term, the government granted two pieces of crown land to elites, encouraging them to start a public toilet business. This attempt might be associated with higher sickness and mortality rates due to the frequent outbreak of disease in the mid-1860s, as shown in Chap. 3. In providing pro-business measures, Governor J. Bowring (1854–1859) granted a land parcel at Circular Pathway in Sheung Wan to a Tepo called Soong Hing to create a bamboo forest and a public toilet among the Chinese residential area.[116] Soong was appointed as a Tepo in 1858, so it is believed the land was granted to him in either 1858 or 1859.[117] From Soong's will probated in 1867, we know he built the toilet, as well as two houses and the bamboo forest there at his expense.[118] A reference figure in 1876 shows that the construction cost of a government toilet was approximately HK$400.[119] Although we do not know the exact date Soong's toilet was built, the rate book shows that a public toilet was registered at 38 circular pathways in 1865.[120]

Following Soong Hing, in 1867, another piece of land at Ship Street in Wanchai was granted to Pang Wa, a building contractor, to establish a privately owned public toilet that came to operate for four decades.[121] His son, Pang Kang Iu, continued to operate this toilet (ten seats) after he died in 1883.[122] In the very beginning, there were no government fee toilet providers to operate; however, a monthly tax of HK$0.60 per seat was introduced in 1873.[123] Obviously, these terms were very favorable to the operators, who sustained their services through charging an entrance fee, of which one or two copper cash was paid by each patron.[124] The pangs only paid the monthly fee from 1873 to 1886, after which the fee was discontinued. The land for building a toilet was originally granted by the government to Pang Wa, while since 1893, there was a change in circumstance that the toilet was held under a Squatters' licence, meaning that Pang Kang Iu was required to pay a small sum of annual rent to use the Crown land (for reference, HK$1.2 was paid for a 154 square feet site in Causeway Bay in 1882), and he had to surrender the land to the government upon request within one month of notice.[125] Through these strategies, it is clear that the government intended to minimize its provision of public toilets; however, the result was far from satisfactory, as the number of privately owned toilets remained unchanged at six between 1865 and 1867.[126] Luckily, as mentioned, the number rapidly increased to 22 in 1868, the year that Chinese merchants realized the high profit of night soil in Shunde. The existence of that market set the stage for the capitalist turn of sanitation and the greater involvement of Chinese in urban hygiene, which eventually put public toilet provision into their hands.

Compared to the government's efforts, the development of privately owned toilets was intense. Public toilets had three sources of income: selling night soil, charging entrance fees, and the premium paid for leasing the land at a higher rate than for other land uses. Both privately owned and government-owned public toilets were relatively scarce in the colony, so much so that the number of daily patrons could be as high as 3,000 or 4,000 in a two-storey privately owned toilet with 51 seats.[127] Here, night soil revenue was boosted by intense facility usage. As shown in Table 4.4, in 1899, the number of toilet seats was 689, while the number of Chinese men in Victoria City ranged from 115,154 to 129,396, from 1897 to 1901 (no population number is available for 1899), so the average number of persons per seat was 167–187, a number far too high for maintaining hygienic conditions.[128] Moreover, in seeking greater profit, most toilets were established in Chinese areas such as Sheung Wan, Taipingshan, and Saiyingpun (Fig. 4.4), which were enclaves of poor Chinese men living in tenement houses that lacked domestic toilets, so that more night soil and entrance fees could be collected, meaning the profit of operating privately owned toilets was good.

Table 4.4 Public toilet location by ownership in Victoria City, 1899 (Number of seats)

District	Government-owned	Privately owned	Total
Causeway Bay	2 (24)	0	2 (24)
Wanchai	2 (40)	4 (65)	6 (105)
Admiralty	0	0	0
Central	0	0	0
Sheung Wan	1 (13)	4 (155)	5 (168)
Taipingshan	2 (68)	2 (83)	4 (151)
Saiyingpun	0	7 (196)	7 (196)
Kennedy town	4 (21)	1 (24)	5 (45)
Total	11 (166)	18 (523)	29 (689)

Source Hong Kong Government, 1899: 7. *Note* (1) Districts are arranged from east to the west of Victoria City. (2) The number of toilets and seats shown here is different from that summarized by Hong Kong Government (1899), the author finds the report author had mistakenly calculated the numbers, and based on the evidence shown in that text new numbers have been calculated

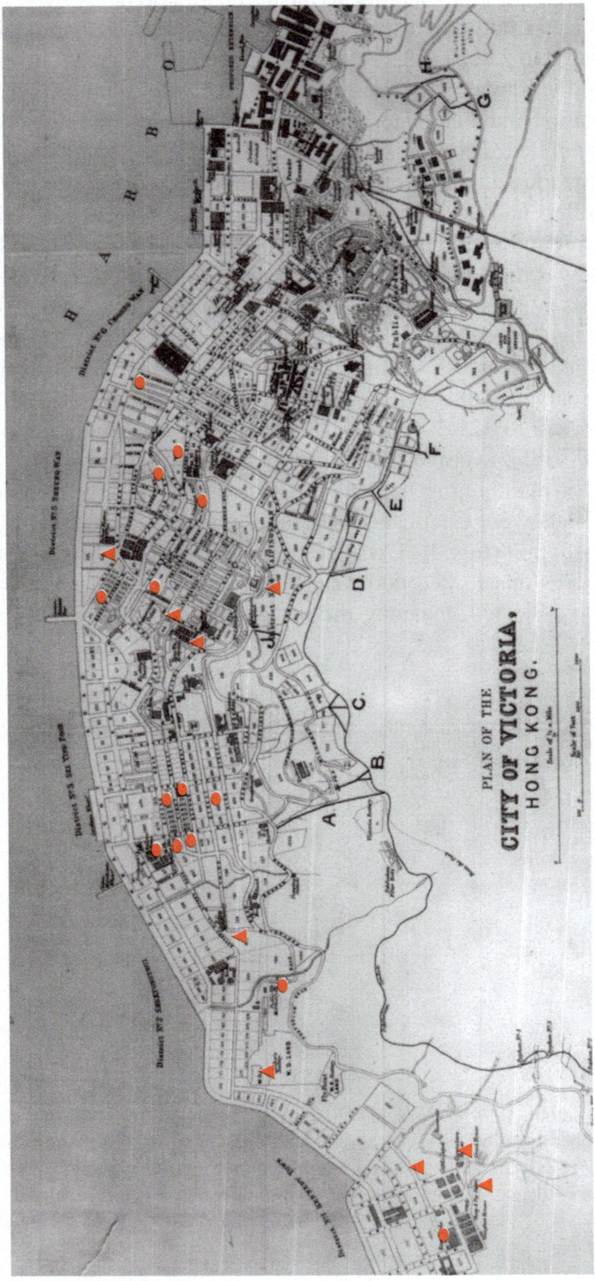

Fig. 4.4 Public Toilet Distribution in the Chinese Quarter of Victoria City, 1899. *Source* The author plotted the distribution by using the following archives: Crown Property, *BB*, 1899; Hong Kong Government, 1899. For the map, Plan of the City of Victoria, CO129/311, 1902, p. 327.
Note ● = Privately owned toilet; ▲ = Government-owned toilet

4.4.3 Higher Rental Return

The profits from selling night soil were good enough to feed a chain of commercial parties; night soil contractors were happy to offer good prices to operators in exchange for the night soil collected in their privately owned toilets; in turn, these operators were willing to pay high rents in exchange for leasing the toilets from the landowners. As Chadwick notes, the real interest was that "these latrines are built and owned by private persons as a business speculation".[129] The good rental return attracted landowners, mainly Chinese, who had the strong market sense to lease out their properties as toilets. The colony's economic structure was based on land investment, whereby the high land price policy created a shortage of available land, which constantly forced rents to increase, as shown in Chap. 2. As a means of production, these toilets were leased to the highest bidder, with returns up to 20% higher than residential development. Combined with the conditions of scarce land, the higher rent was a function of the relative spatial advantages a particular site may have for the collection of night soil, for example, the busyness of the surrounding area. This is shown in how privately owned firms were located and constructed in relation to their external contextual factors and in terms of their internal spatial organization. This not only reflects that toilet landowners made use of external factors to maximize their profit but also reflects that they had an ongoing stake in the particular economic makeup of toilet spaces. In responding to these, they were concerned most with how to maximize the possible toilet gains. Rather than rent being determined by a straightforward equation of supply and demand, services offered and customer visits, Logan and Molotch explain the wider rationale behind rental rates, which depend,

> On the fate of other parcels and those who own and use them... A retailer may depend not only on a substantial number of people nearby but also on a certain type of residential enclave. A Kosher butcher needs Jews; an exclusive boutique needs the trendy rich.[130]

For any consumer business, location is important because more profit can be generated through proximity. Extending this vein, Lefebvre argues that profit depends on a sociospatial matrix of activities and locations.[131] He notes that the production of space is governed by the logic of profit making within a capitalist system; therefore, urban space is produced into a means of production. Urban space is unevenly developed and delineated by its varying specialization of economic functions. It is common knowledge that land supply was extremely limited in nineteenth-century Hong Kong, and this was more of a factor on urban development in the small and densely populated Chinese quarter. It was there that privately owned toilets could succeed particularly well through the use of four spatial strategies that encouraged the frequent use of the toilets, increasing the amount of night soil that could be collected.

First, the toilets were concentrated in the Chinese quarter. Here, there was an enclave of lower-class Chinese living in tenement buildings that lacked domestic toilets (Fig. 4.4). Proximity to the main toilet users was the most important locational advantage of these toilets. As Chadwick notes, "These latrines are large buildings generally standing among or in close proximity to dwellings or shops".[132] Privately owned toilets were located conveniently on either the ground floor or underground within residential areas and were sometimes even adjacent to tenement houses. Such a locational advantage made these toilets easily accessible by their main clients—lower class male Chinese. On the other hand, government public toilets were located distantly from dwellings or within a city block of government buildings to minimize their negative external effects.[133] Second, privately owned toilets were mostly built of brick and two or three stories tall, enabling them to house more toilet seats, increasing night soil collection.[134] The result was that privately owned toilets were located exclusively in the Chinese quarter, where a large number of lower-class Chinese and tenements lacking domestic toilets were concentrated, while the toilets were moderately sized buildings in easily accessible locations of residential areas.

Third is the internal spatial organization of the toilets, the dense layout of the seats inside the building, of which the main goal was the efficient use of space to avoid any wastage of rentable space. The inside of these facilities was basic: "They contain a number of small open-topped compartments with a half-door in front. In each compartment is a sort of seat or rather platform under which is a wooden tub to receive the excreta", notes Chadwick.[135] Having the most seats possible meant being able to serve the most patrons, and so collect more night soil, increasing the property's value. Compared to government toilets, which had approximately ten seats, most privately owned toilets had more than 20 seats.[136] Furthermore, some prominent locations with high footfall, such as 38 circular pathways and 14 Mercer Street, had up to 40 toilet seats.[137] Another large facility at 256 Queen's Road West even had 56 seats,[138] and the building was constructed on a slope so that the upper floor had a second entrance accessible from 29 First Street.

Finally, is the strategy whereby the toilet landowner purchased and owned the properties around their public toilet, establishing a sphere of influence. Public toilets were generally a public nuisance, in particular the strong odor but also public noise and disruption. This could lead to significant complaints being made that could lead to a public toilet being closed down. Therefore, the establishment of a sphere of influence, through purchasing adjacent properties, helped control public complaints about the facility, as the residents near the toilet were also the toilet landowner's tenants. The spheres had the effect of muting local opposition to the issues of living near such poorly maintained public toilets, which was important to both the economic (a means of production) and political (urban regulation) sustainability of these facilities. It was likely that the establishment of the surrounding buffer zones was the key factor that enabled private toilets to operate in the same place for decades (Table 4.6). Meanwhile, government toilets, which lacked such buffer zones, tended to operate for much shorter durations. Controlling the nearby area also allowed for a significant intensification of toilet activities, most notably in the form of having more seats. We shall see the formulation and operation of these spheres in Chap. 5.

These four modes of spatial organization distinguish external contextual factors and internal spatial organization. Combined, they helped increase night soil collection while reducing the risk of complaints being lodged. Their effects also satisfied the operators' needs and concerns, who were therefore more willing to make higher rental bids to operate the facility. The four spatial strategies followed a market agenda to maximize usage at the expense of other concerns; here, then the instrumental use of space played an important role in transforming the toilets into marketable spaces. Obviously, toilet properties were part of a vibrant land market that they were being traded in a relatively sophisticated financial market. Landowners were trying to secure their assets, converting it from something like a business. Some landowners owned more than one toilet property that they leased, and toilet properties were always changing hands (as a standalone purchase or as a package of land). People participated in this market for a variety of financial reasons, sometimes simply to sell for a profit, other times to restructure a greater collection of investments, or to pay off debts due to bankruptcy or financial constraints. Overall, these financial actions shaped a dynamic market for toilet properties. For example, the toilet at 256 Queen's Road West was owned by four different families in seven decades. The property was first held by Kwok Acheong from 1868 until it was sold to Tso Wing Yung in 1873. In the mid-1880s, the Tso family sold it to Hu Tso to clear unpaid debts incurred after the family head died in 1876.[139] Finally, the toilet came under the control of Tang Luk's family at the end of the 1880s, and they held the property until 1925. Another example involves one of the top taxpayers in 1876 and 1881, Ng Sang. Due to his huge losses in the 1881 property crash, as shown in Chap. 2, one of his toilets, located in Rutter Lane, was sold, and the other was forced to close after his death in 1883.

While most of these privately owned toilets were held by a single family or company, a few were held by a partnership. For example, the toilet at 14 Mercer Street was held by Chan Pui and Ku Fai Shan in the early twentieth century.[140] The high exchange value of this toilet can be seen in Chan Pui's will of 1917.[141] In the will, the value of six shops on Tai Wong Street East in Wanchai is HK$6,000, which is less than a single public toilet. He also owned a 40-seat public toilet on Mercer Street in Sheung Wan, which was valued at HK$21,000. These six shops and Mercer Street public toilets were of an equal size and were also in local economic hubs of the time.[142] The high value indicates how private public toilets functioned as sites of capital accumulation; they were definitely prosperous businesses to invest in but needed social and political connections to do so, which will be discussed in Chap. 5.

A 1904 government paper shows the monthly cost of managing a government toilet at Tai Hang village in Causeway Bay, giving an indication of the general costs.[143] The quantity of night soil collected and sold from this toilet was too low to economically sustain its operation, so the operator requested compensation from the government. The total cost was approximately HK$27.3 a month, consisting of a caretaker's salary of HK$10, deodorization (opium packing) and disinfection (coal tarring, Jeyes Fluid and lime washing) for HK$10.3, toilet utensils (lamp oil and brooms) for HK$3, and paying night soil contractors to remove the night soil for HK$4. While the operators of private ones had to pay HK$0.03 for each picul removed from their toilets in 1882,[144] by the 1910s, that charge had risen to HK$0.10 per picul.[145] Compared to government toilets, the operating cost of privately owned toilets was lower. As shown, the government had no power to order toilet operators to deodorize or disinfect the night soil or the toilets, which was the first major cost in government toilets (Table 4.5). The second major cost was the caretaker salary, who

Table 4.5 Income and operating cost of a privately owned public toilet

Income Source	HK$	Expenditure Item	HK$ (per month)
Selling night soil	0.28 per picul	Tax per toilet seat	0.60 (at least 20 seats per toilet)
Entrance fee	0.01–0.02 per patron (approximately 4,000 patrons in a toilet situated in the Central)	A caretaker salary	7–10
		Lamp oil, brooms	3
		Night soil removal fee	0.03–0.10 per picul
		Rent	20 percent higher than residential rent

Source The author compiled the data and information from the text

was employed to receive the fee from patrons, which allowed the actual operator to visit the toilets to supervise the business only about once a day. Overall, privately owned toilets were operated cheaply. Being able to operate so cheaply certainly increased the incentives to continue operating toilet services.

4.5 The Vibrant Night Soil Market and Public Toilets

From the early twentieth century onwards, when the world silk market entered a downturn that damaged night soil demand in China, pail public toilets (both government-owned and privately owned) were no longer economically viable. In the first and second decades, the Pearl River Delta was frequently devastated by floods, reducing the night soil demand for the cultivation of mulberry trees. Worse still, night soil contractors would be unable to collect debts from farmers (the night soil was paid for after the harvest) and consequently suffer significant financial losses.[146] Therefore, the fees paid by contractors to the government decreased significantly, so that government night soil revenue, including scavenging revenue, was HK$52,200 in 1903, a 23 percent drop compared to the previous year.[147] Three years later, the figure further dropped to HK$41,685, approximately 0.5 percent of the total budget yearly revenue. From the early 1900s onwards, night soil revenue was in constant decline, and the percentage of total revenue remained below one percent.

In addition to natural disasters, dangerous shipping routes and political turmoil posed more threats to the night soil business. In 1915, pirates often controlled the channel from Bocca Tigris to night soil depots at Wong Lin in Shunde, the destination for Hong Kong night soil. They ransomed the night soil contractors for large sums of money by threatening to burn the night soil boats and slaughter the crew for any delay of payment. The Chinese government armed launches to escort the boats through the dangerous area, but the contractors were not free from any charges for this. In the subsequent year, the southernmost province, Guangdong (where Shunde is located), declared independence when the first President of China, Yuan Shi Kai, made himself the emperor. This declaration significantly disrupted trade with the region. The depredations of robbers and soi-disant soldiers in the city districts where night soil was sold to mulberry tree growers and the anarchy that prevailed at Wong Lin meant that even if it were possible to transport night soil there, it would not be possible to sell it. This made it difficult for contractors to sell their night soil, and they were forced to dump the night soil in the Hong Kong Sea. Obviously, this rendered fulfilling the government night soil contracts impossible, so contractor payments to the government were greatly reduced. Eventually, the terms of payment actually reversed, with the government having to negotiate with the contractors to remove the night soil at a cost of HK$3,800 a month. This, combined with the loss of night soil revenue, meant that the government took a total monthly revenue reduction of approximately HK$8,000 in 1916.[1]

Due to the disasters and the Chinese silk industry shrinking due to the Great Depression, the amount of land cultivated for mulberry trees, mulberry leaf and silkworm cocoon production, and raw silk exports all registered their first ever decrease in Guangdong since the early 1840s. There was a 67 percent reduction in the above four items between the periods 1925 to 1929 and 1930 to 1934, as Table 4.3 shows. The downward trend of the world silk market diminished the demand for night soil in southern China. This made it difficult to secure toilet operators that would pay a considerable sum to lease privately owned public toilets. Rental returns from public toilets drastically decreased, so investors became less interested and quickly withdrew from the toilet market. Consequently, the number of these toilets decreased significantly from 18 to 13 between 1900 and 1905 and further decreased to eight and two by 1920 and 1930, respectively (Fig. 4.1). This shows the commercial-toilet industry shows how vividly the government-business mode of urban governance was mediated by "toilet economies" that toilet services were impossible to sustain without high night soil prices.

An accumulation of events, kicked off by frequent disease outbreaks, rising pressure from the European business sector, and the downward trend of the world silk market, reshaped the government's approach towards sanitation, leading to a substantial number of government toilets finally being built from 1900 onwards. The annual outbreaks of the plague from 1894 onwards, with persistently high mortality rates of over 90 percent, alarmed the Hong Kong General Chamber of Commerce. In response, the Chamber sent a petition of more than 1,000 signatures to Chamberlain, the Secretary of State for the Colonies in 1901. From an economic perspective, the Chamber argued that the colony's welfare was bound to its sanitary condition, and the key to securing this was to improve the morality of lower-class Chinese in the colony. It therefore recommended the close surveillance of Chinese bodies in urban spaces. As such, one focus was the government acquisition of privately owned toilets and the investment of public funds in the construction of additional government toilets. This caught the attention of the British imperial government, and high pressure from there prompted the colonial government to accelerate the construction of new government public toilets. Specifically, the construction of the fourteen public toilets proposed in the 1897 *Latrine Ordinance* was carried out rapidly in the early twentieth century.

The pail system was gradually retired when water flush toilets, in the form of troughs, were introduced in underground government public toilets in the early 1910s (Table 4.6).

4.6 Conclusion

Through night soil, the economic sustainability of Hong Kong's public toilets was connected to China's silk industry and the global consumer silk market. Public toilets were imbricated in the world system of peripheral areas supplying resources (night soil) to semiperipheral areas (China) for use in silk production, which supplied colonial core economies. The high demand for Hong Kong night soil was well timed with the opening of China after the First Opium War, which led to the further incorporation of Delta's silk industry into the world silk economy. This meant that night soil demand was tied to European and United States silk demand. The emergence of economic links between the Chinese silk industry, the China-Hong Kong cross border night soil business, and the Hong Kong land market in the late 1860s drove the development of a citywide network of public toilets, both government-owned and privately owned, that served as night soil collection points to support the colony's economic interests and sanitation needs. Under these circumstances, toilet provision was exposed to global economic restructuring. Therefore, the economic sustainability and rationale of the toilet services was highly dependent on the dynamics of this economic restructuring.

A major feature of public toilet provision was the dominance of commercial toilets (both government-owned and privately owned), with a pronounced capitalist character in terms of their quasi-commercial management. The bulk of these toilets were operated by Chinese businesses, especially landowners, who entered the toilet market to lease their property as toilets for the collection of night soil. The toilet economies of privately owned toilets, consisting of night soil sales, entrance fees, and land rental to private toilets, generated gains above typical urban land uses, such as housing. The economic awareness of certain resourceful Chinese, especially landowners, meant that they developed new business opportunities while taking up new roles as public service providers. Ultimately, their efforts contributed to a mode of shared governance of daily public health in the colony. This facilitated the colonial government to offer pro-business measures for public toilets, and in turn, the Chinese worked with the government in commodifying toilet provision into a means of production. In doing so, the Chinese relationship with the government was restructured, and in providing toilets, they became partners with the government, especially in the context of a very limited land supply and concern about poor sanitation. The toilets effectively being night soil collection points meant that they were inevitably seen as marketable public space, which contrasted sharply with the idea of toilets as merely moralizing spaces. The toilets nonetheless supplied a critical boost to government and Chinese revenue while bluntly solving the lower class Chinese's public defecation problem. Appearing out of the colonial order, a spatial order shaped by the capitalist

Table 4.6 Privately owned toilets in Victoria City and their owners, 1865–1930

Toilet site (Seat no.)	Year (Total toilet no.)												
	1865 (6)	1868 (22)	1870 (20)	1877 (18)	1882 (20)	1888 (19)	1892 (17)	1895 (22)	1899 (18)	1905 (14)	1912 (12)	1920 (8)	1925 (7)	1930 (2)
Belcher Street (24)									Unclear	Unclear	Hsui Oi Tong			
20 Caine Road		Lun Teen Wah	Sunteen Who											
50 Center Street (28)					Kwok Acheong's Estate	Kwok's Estate	Kwok's Estate	Kwok's Estate	Unclear	Mrs. Katie. David	Mrs. Katie David			
1 Chee Chee Lane (Near Po Hing Fong)		Pang Wa	Pang Wa											

(continued)

Table 4.6 (continued)

Toilet site (Seat no.)	Year (Total toilet no.)													
	1865 (6)	1868 (22)	1870 (20)	1877 (18)	1882 (20)	1888 (19)	1892 (17)	1895 (22)	1899 (18)	1905 (14)	1912 (12)	1920 (8)	1925 (7)	1930 (2)
10 Cheung Kang Lane (Now Dominion Center, Wanchai)					Rev G. Burno									
2 Chu Tsze Lane (located in Sheung Wan)				Pang Wa	Pang Wa	Pang's Estate								
38 Circular Pathway (40)	Soong Hing	Soong's Estate	Soong's Estate	Soong's Estate	Tang Luk	Tang's Estate	Tang's Estate	Tang's Estate	Tang's Estate	Tang's Estate	Tang's Estate	Tang's Estate	Tang's Estate	
Connaught Road							Lo In-wa							
116 Des Voeux Road Central (48)		Choy Hing	Choy Hing	Choy Hing	Choy Chan	Choy Chan	Choy Chan	Choy Chan	Choy Chan	Choy's Estate	Choy's Estate			
Des Voeux Road West	Kwong Yune													
46 Eastern Street			Wong A Shing	Kwok Acheong										

(continued)

Table 4.6 (continued)

Toilet site (Seat no.)	Year (Total toilet no.)													
	1865 (6)	1868 (22)	1870 (20)	1877 (18)	1882 (20)	1888 (19)	1892 (17)	1895 (22)	1899 (18)	1905 (14)	1912 (12)	1920 (8)	1925 (7)	1930 (2)
82–84 First Street (48)								Hu Tso	Hu Tso	Lo Kun Ting	Lo Kun Ting	Tang Mui	Tang Mui	
2 Gough Street (27)							Chan Pui	Chan Pui	Chan Pui	Chan Pui	Chan Pui	Chan Pui		
3 Heung Hing Lane (42)		Tso Wing Yung	Lee A Lok	Lo Fat Yuen	Lo Fat Yuen	Wong I Lung	Wong I Lung	Wong I Lung	Wong's Estate	Wong's Estate	Wong's Estate			
23 High Street								Pang Wa's Estate						
28 Hill Road (Previous number 12 Tung Wo Lane East) (8)		Bw Ming Chow Tong	Chiu Yun	Cheong Yuk Shang	Cheong Yuk Shang	Cheong Yuk Shang	Unclear	Unclear	Unclear					
192 Hollywood Road						Leroiow								

(continued)

Table 4.6 (continued)

Toilet site (Seat no.)	Year (Total toilet no.)													
	1865 (6)	1868 (22)	1870 (20)	1877 (18)	1882 (20)	1888 (19)	1892 (17)	1895 (22)	1899 (18)	1905 (14)	1912 (12)	1920 (8)	1925 (7)	1930 (2)
12 Kennedy Street (20)		Chung Lo Luey	Chung Lo Luey	Lo Iu Wa	Lo Iu Wa	Lo Iu Wa	Lo Iu Wa	Lo Iu Wa	Lo Iu Wa					
3 Lok Ku Road (Previous number 23 West Street)								Pung Tai Un						
2 Market Street (now Po Hing Fong)		Cheong A Ssow												
3 Market Street (as above)	Cheong A Choy	Rde Rozario	Kwok Acheong											
32 Market Street (as above)								Hu Tso						
14 Mercer Street (40)			How A Shun	Lau Ting	Cheng Sing Yeung	Unclear	Li Hiung	Chan Pui	Chan Pui	Chan Pui	Chan Pui + Ku Fai Shan	Chan's estate + Ku Fai Shan	Yeung Ho	

(continued)

Table 4.6 (continued)

Toilet site (Seat no.)	Year (Total toilet no.)													
	1865 (6)	1868 (22)	1870 (20)	1877 (18)	1882 (20)	1888 (19)	1892 (17)	1895 (22)	1899 (18)	1905 (14)	1912 (12)	1920 (8)	1925 (7)	1930 (2)
12 On Ning Lane (19)					Tso Wing Yung's Estate	Tso's Estate	Tso's Estate	Tso's Estate	Unclear	Chan Pui	Chan Pui	Mak To Hung	Ho To Hang	Lau Tsuin Kwai
2 Po Yan Street (Previous name Cemetery Street)			Ly Sne Guong											
5 Po Yan Street (as above)	Tsig Kee	Unclear	Siemssen											
1 Pound Lane (41)		Kwok Acheong	Kwok Acheong	Kwok Acheong	Ho Tsim	Ng Ping Sam	Ng Ping Sam	Ng Ping Sam	Unclear					
8 Pound Lane		Lum Tun Kee												
25 Pound Lane		Lum Tun Kee												

(continued)

Table 4.6 (continued)

Toilet site (Seat no.)	Year (Total toilet no.)												
	1865 (6)	1868 (22)	1870 (20)	1877 (18)	1882 (20)	1888 (19)	1892 (17)	1895 (22)	1899 (18)	1905 (14)	1912 (12)	1920 (8)	1925 (7)	1930 (2)
256 Queen's Road West (56) (could be accessed from 29 First Street)		Kwok Acheong	Kwok + Tso Wing Yuug	Tso's Estate	Tso's Estate	Hu Tso	Tang Luk's Estate	Tang's Estate	Tang's Estate	Tang's Estate	Tang' Estate	Tang's Estate	Tang's Estate	
1 Rutter Lane (now Po Hing Mansion)		Unclear	Ng Sang	Ng Sang	Ng Sang	Pow Ping Kwan	Li Tung Shan	Chan Pui						
5 Rutter Lane (as above)		A Fow	Ng Sang	Ng Sang	Ng Sang									
8 Sai On Lane				Chor Tak Ki										
3 Sam To Lane (16)				Ng Sang	Chung Shui Hung	Ip Ching Chuen	Ip's Estate	Ip's Estate	Ip's Estate	Ip's Estate	Ip's Estate	Ip's Estate	Tsung Po Land Sweet	Tsung Po Land Sweet

(continued)

Table 4.6 (continued)

Toilet site (Seat no.)	Year (Total toilet no.)													
	1865 (6)	1868 (22)	1870 (20)	1877 (18)	1882 (20)	1888 (19)	1892 (17)	1895 (22)	1899 (18)	1905 (14)	1912 (12)	1920 (8)	1925 (7)	1930 (2)
89 s Street				Yun leo	Tsui Cheong Lung	Tsui Cheong Lung								
113 s Street (23)							Tsui Cheong Lung	Lui Shung	Unclear					
23 Ship Street (10)		Pang Wa	Pang Wa	Pang Wa	Pang Wa	Pang's Estate	Pang's Estate	Pang's Estate	Pang's Estate	Pang's Estate				
Ship Street Back Lane	Choy Hoam													
30 Stone Nullah (26)					Tso Po To	Tso Po To	Tso Po To	Tso Po To	Tso Po To	Tso Po To	Tso Po To	Tang Luk's Estate	Tang's Estate	
13 Tai Wong Street West (9)					Jardine Matheson	Jardine Matheson	Jardine Matheson	Jardine Matheson	Unclear					
6 Tak Hing Alley East (near now Ham Yu Street)	Hoong Chaong	Hoong Chaong	Siemssen	Siemssen	Siemssen	Siemssen	Siemssen	Siemssen						

(continued)

Table 4.6 (continued)

Toilet site (Seat no.)	Year (Total toilet no.)													
	1865 (6)	1868 (22)	1870 (20)	1877 (18)	1882 (20)	1888 (19)	1892 (17)	1895 (22)	1899 (18)	1905 (14)	1912 (12)	1920 (8)	1925 (7)	1930 (2)
2 Tun Wo Street		Unclear												
60 Tung Street (Previous name East Street)		Lum Fo Yow Tong	Lum Fo Yow Tong											
57 Wanchai Road		Cheep Yuen	Cheep Yuen	Tsap Who Tong										
2 West Street (Now Hua Qin Building, Sheung Wan)		Cheong A Ssow												

Source Hong Kong Government, 1899; HKRS38-2, *RB*, 1865–1930.
Note (1) Seat numbers were recorded in 1899; empty cell indicates facility closure

system and a discursive moral order of Otherness was manifested. This does not mean though that capitalist logic overtook moral logic or that the government was moral and business was just; rather, it represents that government and business, as well as capitalist and moral logics, had become interdependent. In the next chapter, we will see the negotiated relationship between government and business and the negotiated meaning between morality and capitalism that existed within the public toilets, which together led to the formation of a new moral geography.

Notes

1. HKRS38-2-4, 38–2-5, *RB*, 1867, 1868.
2. Eng, 1986; So, 1986.
3. Eng, 1986; Wong; 2017.
4. Li, 1981: 71.
5. Eng, 1986: 35; So, 1986: 83.
6. Eng, 1986: 35.
7. Wong, 2017: 164.
8. Eng, 1986; So, 1986.
9. So, 1986: 83. For the value of teal, see Yan, 2015: ix.
10. Wong, 2017: 636.
11. Eng, 1986: 42; So, 1986: 83.
12. Eng, 1986: 41.
13. Guangdong Province Chorography, 2004: 275.
14. Wong, 2017: 361–2.
15. Wong, 2017: 361–2.
16. So, 1986: 77; Wong, 2017: 262–6.
17. So, 1986: 83–4; Wong, 2017: 361–2.
18. So, 1986: 80.
19. Guangzhou City Chorography Office, 1995: 83; Lau, 2006: 68; Wong, 2017: 224.
20. Eng, 1986; Li, 1981; So, 1986; Wong, 2017.
21. Eng, 1986: 36.
22. Wong, 2017: 164.
23. Eng, 1986: 36.
24. Wong, 2017: 230.
25. Eng, 1986: 39.
26. Wong, 2017: 237.
27. Lau, 2006: 326.
28. Wong, 2017: 220.
29. Lau, 2006: 172.
30. Wong, 2017: 170.
31. Eng, 1986: 44.
32. Wong, 2017: 16. For the value of Haikwan tael, see Yan, 2015: ix.
33. Lau, 2006: 66.
34. Eng, 1986; So, 1986; Wong, 2017.

35. Eng, 1986: 53, 60; Wong, 2017: 172.
36. Guangdong Province Chorography, 2004: 282–3.
37. Hui, 1994: 72.
38. Eng, 1986: 101.
39. Howard quote in So, 1986: 78.
40. So, 1986: 116.
41. Lau, 2006: 171–4, 316–29.
42. Lau, 2006: 327; Wong, 2017: 553.
43. Wong, 2017: 649.
44. So, 1986: 136.
45. For Western silk import, see Wong, 2017: 716–20.
46. Shen, 1936.
47. Ferguson, 2014; King, 1911; Li, 1999; Xue, 2005.
48. Ferguson, 2014: 391.
49. Li, 1999: 32–5.
50. Registration of Persons Ordinance, https://oelawhk.lib.hku.hk/items/show/1988 (accessed 10 September 2020).
51. Xue, 2005: 47–58.
52. According to Google Map.
53. Chadwick, 1882: 21.
54. Hong Kong Government, 1899: 6.
55. CRN, HKRS149- 2–534, 1869.
56. CRN, HKRS149- 2–534, 1869.
57. CRN, HKRS149- 2–534, 1869.
58. CRN, HKRS149-2–1245, 1885.
59. Xue, 2005: 43.
60. Evans, 1987; Melosi, 2005; Wohl, 1983.
61. Macpherson, 1987; Rogaski, 2004; Yu, 2003.
62. CRN, HKRS149-2–581, 1870.
63. CRN, HKRS149-2–688, 1872.
64. CRN, HKRS149-2–1883, 1898.
65. CRN, HKRS149-2–1883, 1898; PLK Archive; TWH, 1970: 66.
66. CRN, HKRS149-2–1415, 1889.
67. For the Chamber, see CS/I002/00013571.GIF, CS/I018/00174441.GIF, Carl Smith Collection. For the JP appointment, see Justices of Peace, *GG*, 3 June 1902, p.932, 4 March 1907, p. 342.
68. CRN, HKRS149-2–1415, 1889.
69. The Bribery Charges, *SCMP*, 24 August 1906, The ownership of this toilet refers to Table 4.6.
70. CRN, HKRS149-2–1245; 149–2-1247; 149–2-1251; 149–2-1374; 149–2-1375.
71. CRN, HKRS149-2–1415, 1889; Slaughter House Farm, HKRS149-2–1123, 1884.
72. Sanitary Superintendent's Report, *SP*, 1890.
73. Symons, 1996: 5.

74. Night Soil Contracts, *BB*, 1887–1903.
75. CRN, HKRS149-2–1181, 1885.
76. Conservancy Contracts, *BB*, 1904–30.
77. Latrine Accommodation, CO129/299, 1901, p. 298–302.
78. Crown Property, *BB*, 1891, F6-7.
79. Crown property, 1891, F6-7; CRN, HKRS149-2–1247, 1885.
80. CRN, HKRS149-2–1247, 1885.
81. Crown Property, *BB*, 1891–99.
82. Latrine Accommodation, CO129/299, 1901, p. 298–302.
83. Ordinance for the Maintenance of Order and Cleanliness, *GG*, 22 June 1867, No.96, p. 231–2.
84. Hong Kong Government, 1899.
85. Chadwick, 1882: 20.
86. Hong Kong Government, 1899: 3.
87. Additional by-laws, *GG*, 8 December 1894, p. 1054; By-laws under Public Health and Buildings Ordinance, 1903–1909, *GG*, 29 September 1912, p. 565.
88. Report of the Secretary, Sanitary Board, for 1896, *SP*, 1897, p. 343–44.
89. CRN, HK149-2–1181, 1885.
90. By-laws under the Public Health and Buildings Ordinance, 1903–1909, *GG*, 22 September 1912, p. 565–7.
91. Chadwick, 1882:18.
92. CRN, HKRS149-2–1181, 1885.
93. CRN, HKRS149-2–1181, 1885.
94. CRN, HKRS149-2–1181, 1885.
95. CRN, HKRS149-2–1251, 1885. More regulations to supervise the works of contractors, see By-laws under the Public Health Ordinance, 1887, *GG*, 23 November 1889, p.919, 30 November 1889, p. 984; By-laws under the Public Health and Buildings Ordinance, 1903–1909, *GG*, 22 September 1912, p.565–7.
96. Chadwick, 1882:23. 1 ton equals to 16.53 piculs.
97. Hong Kong Government, 1899: 5.
98. Population, *BB*, 1897, M2.
99. Macpherson, 1987; Rogaski, 2004; Yu, 2010.
100. Xue, 2005: 60.
101. CRN, HKRS149-2–581, 1870; HKRS38-2–40, *RB*, 1882.
102. Contract for the general surface scavenging, HKRS149-2–1595; Contract for the Removal of Excretal Matters, HKRS149-2–1415, 1889; Sanitary Superintendent's Report, *SP*, 1890; Slaughter House Farm, HKRS 149–2-1123, 1884.
103. Alleged Bribery of Public Servant, *SCMP*, 23 August 1906; the Bribery Charges, *SCMP*, 24 August 1906; Alleged Bribery, *SCMP*, 25 October 1906. Additionally, refers to Table 4.6. However, the toilet at Gough Street was registered under Chan's name in the rate book, other evidence (the above newspapers and Ng Tat Chi v. Chan Pui, *HKWP*, 2 January 1896) shows the toilet was leased, but the identity of the toilet landowner is unclear.

104. Ibid.
105. HKRS38-2–23, 38–2-33, 38–2-57, 38–2-81, *RB*, 1877, 1880, 1888, 1895.
106. AJPH, *GG*, 11 February 1882, p. 82.
107. Ibid.
108. For the will, see Choy Chan, HKRS144-4–1772, 1905; Ip Ching Chuen, HKRS144-4–764, 1888; Tang Luk, HKRS144-4–680, 1887; Tsoo Wing Yung, HKRS144-4-338, 1876. More about Tso's will, see Tso Sum Cho and Others v. Tso lai Tong and Another, *HKDP*, 30 September 1885; and Choy's will, see A Disputed Will, *HKDP*, 27 June 1905. For the estate, see Probate, *BB*, 1876–1905. For Kwok's estate, see Smith, 1971. For Ip's estate, see CS/I002/00017229.GIF, Carl Smith Collection.
109. CS/I001/00009949.GIF, CS/I001/00009950.GIF, Carl Smith Collection; Justices of Peace, GG, 4 March 1904, p.342; PLK Archive; TWH, 1907: 65.
110. Choy Chan, HKRS144-4–1772, 1905; CS/I005/00043257.GIF, CS/I005/00043259.GIF, Carl Smith Collection; PLK Archive; Probate, *BB*, 1905; TWH, 1970: 66.
111. Chadwick, 1882: 55.
112. Revenue, Governor Sir H. Robinson to Sir F. Rogers, Bart, 21 May 1863. Enclosure 3 in No. 3, *BPP 1863–1881*, Vol. 25, 1971, p.7.
113. Bristow, 1984: 27.
114. CS/I018/00178042.GIF, Carl Smith Collection; Chan, 1991; Munn, 2009: 123.
115. Lindblom, 1977.
116. Soong Hing, HKRS144-4–180, 1867.
117. CS/I004/00039419.GIF, Carl Smith Collection.
118. Soong Hing, HKRS144-4–180, 1867.
119. Payments, *LC*, 6 March 1876, 1876.
120. HKRS38-2–3, *RB*, 1865. Rate books before 1865 did not include the function of the properties, therefore it is possible the toilet might have existed prior to 1865.
121. Latrine at Ship Street, HKRS58-1–14 (98), 1899; Government Latrine at the Upper End of Ship Street, HKRS202-1–13, 1904.
122. Schedule of Taxes, *BB*, 1879, A2; Latrine at Ship Street, HKRS58-1–14-98, 1899; Government Latrine at the Upper End of Ship Street, HKRS202-1–13, 1904.
123. Schedule of Taxes, *BB*, 1883: A2.
124. Chadwick, 1882: 18; Hong Kong Government, 1899: 2.
125. Squatters' Licences, *GG*, 21 January 1882, No. 16, p.29.
126. HKRS38-2–3, HKR 38–2-4, *RB*, 1865, 1867.
127. Chadwick, 1882: 18.
128. Population, *BB*, 1897, M2, 1901, M2.
129. Chadwick, 1882: 18.
130. Logan and Molotch, 1987: 21, 24.
131. Lefebvre, 1991.

132. Chadwick, 1882: 18.
133. Crown Property, *BB*, 1891–1911.
134. Chadwick, 1882: 18; Hong Kong Government, 1899: 8–10; Public Latrines in Hong Kong, *HKT*, 26 March 1891.
135. Chadwick. 1882: 18.
136. Hong Kong Government, 1899: 8–10.
137. Hong Kong Government, 1899: 7.
138. Hong Kong Government, 1899: 9.
139. For the transfer from Kwok to Tso, see Quok A Cheong to Tsoo Wing Yung, HKRS205-11A-887–5, 1873. More about Tso, see *HKDP*, 30 September 1885. It is not sure if Tso was connected with Tso Wing Chow, the brother of Tso Yau. The latter was the father of Tso Seen Wan, a Legislative Councilor in the early twentieth century. See, CS/I005/00044891.GIF, CS/I005/00044892.GIF, Carl Smith Collection.
140. HKRS38-2–122, *RB*, 1912; HKRS38-2–140, *RB*, 1918.
141. Chan Pui, HKRS144-4–3130, 1918.
142. The toilet seat refers to Table 4.5. More or less, the area could be calculated from the crown rent, as stated in the rate book, see HKRS38-2–137, *RB*, 1917.
143. Public Latrine at Tai Hang Village, HKRS202-1–13, 1904.
144. Chadwick, 1882: 18; CRN, HKRS 149–2-1181, 1885.
145. CRN, HKRS1149-2–3172, 1912; By-laws under the Public Health and Buildings Ordinance, 1903–1909, *GG*, 22 September 1912, p.566.
146. Report of the Head of the Sanitary Department, *AR*, 1915, M6 and 1916, M5-6.
147. Conservancy Contracts, *BB*, 1903; Nightsoil Contracts, *BB*, 1902.

Chapter 5
A Blending of Moral and Capitalist Logics in Public Toilets

5.1 Overview

Public toilets were part of a moral project that originated from the Hong Kong colonial government, as such they were a technology to regulate lower-class Chinese in terms of how they relieve their daily needs. Imbricated with the moral project was an effort to neutralize the perceived health risks of lower-class Chinese and dense living conditions to urban space. What eventuated in practice was a citywide network of public toilets, whereby both government-owned and privately owned toilets came to operate primarily as night soil collection points. This occurred under the influence of various economic links and markets, namely, the local night soil and land markets, the regional silk production industry, and the world consumer silk market. As a business venture, the most important aim of public toilet proprietors was to maintain night soil manurial value. This was critical for the economic sustainability of toilet services and required strategies to maintain toilet cleanliness, which concerned both capitalistic and moralistic concerns. Sometimes poorly maintained, located in dense residential areas, and lacking thorough deodorization measures for the night soil to preserve manurial value, it was difficult for public toilets not to be a public nuisance. Nevertheless, these toilets were successfully operated for decades in a densely populated city and did contribute to the maintenance of general sanitation. This arouses the question: how did their operation fulfill moral and capitalist concerns for over half a century, continuing up until the early twentieth century?

In a capitalist economy, conflicts emerge between urban space as a means of production to generate profit and the resulting urban growth that quickly worsens living conditions and even property values themselves, such as poor sanitation. Relieving sanitation problems require the establishment of urban orders in the form of cleanliness through the regulation of space, but this process can threaten the profit accumulation process. Based on empirical studies, it is argued that the public toilets in nineteenth century Hong Kong became overlapping moral-economic spaces, led by efforts of both the government and Chinese business. In these moral-economic spaces, the goals of profit accumulation and the regulation of space were blended

Y. Chong, *Toilet as Business for the Hygiene of the Chinese Community in Colonial Hong Kong*, https://doi.org/10.1007/978-981-19-1396-9_5

together, albeit mediated by toilet economies (night soil sales, entrance fees, and privately owned toilet rental) and regulation. As Polanyi argues, "regulation and markets, in effect, grew up together".[1] Under a more restrictive mercantile system, markets are highly developed, but they are subject to significant institutional regulations that aimed to safeguard the state treasury instead of developing out of a market dynamic of profit. It should also be emphasized that regulation is central to developing markets in a way that can support capitalist competition. From these two angles, we see how markets interacting with regulation turn them interdependent on each other.

Following this logic, we will see how the Hong Kong public toilet market was constructed by regulation. Operating in a quasi-commercial mode, both government-owned and privately owned toilets functioned as sanitation infrastructure under the regulation of the court and an on-site inspection system, which monitored toilet conditions and night soil removal. By highlighting the role of business and the combined effects of state regulation and markets in maintaining urban hygiene, the author hopes to avoid the one-sided conventional assumption that public health merely rests upon the efforts of the colonial government. Efforts to improve hygiene could not simply rely on the government, either through state coercion or surveillance but also the Chinese business elites' collaboration through the market economy, guided by toilet economies and land interests.

It is worth noting that the availability and viability of commercial toilets (both government-owned and privately owned toilets were operated in a quasi-commercial mode) helped maintain urban hygiene, which was an index of morality. The result had political consequences for colonial government-Chinese business relations, and ultimately, the distinction between morality and capitalism, as well as the spatial relation between colonizer and colonized, came to be negotiated in public toilets. While the contradictory needs of securing economic value and improving public health posed practical challenges in managing the toilets, they also prompted the production of a new urban order that could satisfy these competing agendas. This had important impacts on the formation of a new moral geography that pushed capitalist concern to operate within toilets and sanitation more generally. Thus, this chapter first identifies the regulatory measures (regulations, human and nonhuman inspection systems) employed by the colonial government and then the economic (sphere of influence) and social (social networks) strategies used by Chinese business elites to ensure both urban hygiene and profit. The task here is to unravel the complex interplay between colonizer and colonized, race and class, regulation and market, as well as the moral and capitalist logics in the toilets and the regulation of urban space.

5.2 Government: Surveillance and Regulation

Public toilets not only had practical purposes to maintain urban hygiene but also discursive purposes that they had moral effects, such as conditioning self-regulating sanitary behaviors among people (toilet users, toilet operators and night soil contractors), which could safeguard urban order.[2] The central tenet was to internalize proper behaviors, such as not defecating in public and, more importantly, maintaining toilet cleanliness and removing night soil from toilets without polluting the neighborhood. This approach to disciplining behaviour and developing responsibility for maintaining urban hygiene rested on self-regulation rather than external constraints and legal regulation.

Embedded in racial politics, Chinese were depicted by the colonial government as morally low and therefore ignorant of public health. Furthermore, this meant it was believed that the development of self-regulation of sanitary behaviour among Chinese would be a slow process, and it was this belief that justified the imposition of law on Chinese rather than simply based on their self-regulation.[3] Part of this prejudice against the morality of Chinese arose from the belief that they were only interested in obtaining profits stemming from "toilet economies", without ensuring that the toilet service was carried out expeditiously and with regard to public health.[4] To capture their dynamic relations in regulating urban space in such a context, this study seeks a way of looking at public toilet provisions within a political economy framework. The government compromised profit and night soil odor and chose to work with the Chinese business elites, interplaying political and economic strategies, towards the aim of sustaining toilet services and securing toilet profit.

5.2.1 Compromise of Odor and Profit

The government was very much concerned with the lower-class Chinese population, who defecated in public areas, making their spaces susceptible to the spread of disease in the colony. Therefore, the most effective place to concentrate government public toilets was the Chinese quarter, as shown in Chap. 4, to solve the sanitation issues that only this class of Chinese experienced. Chinese business provided the bulk of privately owned toilets in the quarter, where tenement buildings lacked toilets, so that more night soil could be collected and sold. Moreover, a clean neighbourhood was key to maintaining property values, spurring Chinese landowners to contain bodily waste within public toilets.

The result was a toilet landscape concentrated in the Chinese quarter. Such a concentration mediated how lower class Chinese people used urban space, meaning that the toilets fulfilled a moral imperative, fitting well with the notion of colonial urbanism. This notion shaped the local space as peripheral and already disease ridden and as a site requiring colonial disciplinary power through producing moral geography. This is similar to what Mitchell remarks: that colonial landscapes were the 'world-as-exhibition', which were exhibited as a place of discipline under colonial control.[5] A discursive moral order of urban hygiene was then achieved through the everyday metaphor of colonial discipline over urban space; this was done even though the toilets were mostly offered by Chinese business. Such developments were urgently needed in the quickly growing city, as the amount of agricultural land was greatly diminishing and night soil accumulated in parallel. Here then, toilet economies were crucial.

Whether government or privately owned, both types of toilets used the pail system, whereby keeping the manurial value of the night soil was a strong incentive to ensure that the pails were promptly emptied, a critical practice for a sustainable toilet service. The viability of such a service for lower-class Chinese introduced public health concepts to them, which helped discipline their sanitary behavior. However, if the night soil was diluted with deodorizing or disinfecting substances, it would no longer be worth transporting to the silk production areas in the Pearl River Delta. Without night soil profits, the citywide network of public toilets would not only vanish but also incur a great expense to secure proper night soil disposal. The absence of suitable agricultural land rendered disposing of night soil an almost insurmountable difficulty for the tiny and already highly urbanized colony. To preserve manurial value, neither deodorizing nor disinfecting chemicals were applied to the night soil deposited in the toilets.[6] The government would disinfect night soil in its public toilets during disease outbreaks; however, it had no power to disinfect that deposited in private ones, as it was private property of the toilet operators.[7]

Without proper measures taken to disinfect the night soil, both government-owned and privately owned toilets would generate foul odor and breed diseases and thus became one of the most dangerous sources of infection in the populous Chinese quarter. Rather than remedying the nuisance and combating disease, the most offensive and unwholesome nuisances were always generated by pail public toilets. This type of toilet had a noxious nature, as the night soil was kept in buckets for a whole day and would begin to decompose, therefore giving off miasma and breeding harmful bacteria. To increase the night soil collecting capacity, as noted in Chap. 4, there were approximately twenty toilet seats in an average privately owned public toilet, while there would be approximately ten in government a toilet. Night soil decomposition commences after approximately 12 h and may become harmful after 24–36 h, especially in tropical climates such as Hong Kong.[8] Without disinfection, night soil that has been sitting in public toilets the whole day, the ample oxygen and moisture that facilitated the growth of bacteria created a public nuisance. The insanitary condition of the toilets was well reflected in their noisome odor, which constantly permeated the air in the toilets and the surrounding neighborhood. For example, on account of the repeated complaints about the miasma by people in the vicinity, the windows of a government toilet located at 236 Hollywood Road in the Taipingshan area were kept closed to mitigate the nuisance.[9]

Furthermore, the nuisances were heightened by poor toilet design and construction. As Chadwick observed, the poor design sharpened any negative effects, and the sanitation condition deteriorated sharply in the toilets, that.

> In each compartment is a sort of seat or rather platform under which is a wooden tub to receive the excreta… In one [privately owned toilet], the seats are on the upper floor, sheet metal shoots leading down [the excreta] to the tubs on the floor below, an objectionable arrangement, for there is no means of cleaning the shoots. On the whole the existing latrines are offensive and a nuisance, both as to position and construction, and they are so crowded as to render improvements as to maintenance very difficult.[10]

Furthermore, some toilets were accessed by narrow lanes from the street and so were deep in the city block surrounded by houses. This further blocked ventilation and daylight, trapping the foul air of the toilets. For example, a private toilet at 256 Queen's Road West, owned by the Tang Luk family, was described,

> [The] Brick building is in bad repair practically surrounded by houses, entrance is by 3'0" lane from Queen's Road West and similar entrance from First Street. The latrine is 17'0" below level of First Street. Light and ventilation are bad, foot-rests are of tiles on brick-work, surface is of cement in bad condition, channels to square-lined cesspool.[11]

The poor state of public toilets meant that finding a toilet site was a challenge in such a dense urban landscape. At a Legislative Council meeting in 1902, the Attorney General pointed out the difficulty of finding a site that,

> when, however, the government takes energetic action to meet the wishes of the community by endeavoring to carry out the recommendations of the Sanitary Board with regard to latrines, it is at once opposed by the landowners in the vicinity... This question is not a new one. Everyone knows that latrines are not specially pleasant things to talk about, or to see, nor are they agreeable to one's sense of smell; but in the peculiar conditions of Hong Kong they are absolute necessities.[12]

Indeed, it was impossible to select a site for a pail public toilet anywhere within an inhabited area without causing significant detriment to some of the public. To minimize the effects of miasma, the colonial government was particularly concerned with the time that night soil was removed from the toilets. Based on a study of British practice and experience gained in other tropical colonies as mentioned earlier, it was known that decomposition of night soil took place after 12 h, and it generated its strong odor (at the time believed to be the source of disease) after 24 h; thus, it was determined that night soil must be removed at least once every 24 h to be safe. The night soil was exported by conservancy boats flying a naval flag decided by the Sanitary Board. The boats delivered the night soil to Stonecutters Island to be loaded onto the larger conservancy vessels no later than 2 P.M., and the contractors shall be held responsible for any nuisance caused after that hour.[13] To minimize issues caused by night soil exports, the export station was relocated from Stonecutters Island to further west at Tsuen Wan and then Kwai Chung in the 1890s and 1910s, respectively.[14]

Clearly, night soil removal and the insanitary condition of both government-owned and privately owned public toilets were in contrast with the rising belief in a correlation between odor (from night soil or swamps) and disease and the consciousness of cultivating civilization that arose in eighteenth-century Europe.[15] At the time, the first British Sanitary Commissioner, Edwin Chadwick, forwarded the argument that associated diseases with the environment, the belief that all foul smells were also diseases, as noted in Chap. 1.[16] Based on this health logic, an emphasis on the miasmatic effect of pail public toilets generated from night soil was constructed. This posited that disease occurred from exposure to the pathogenic emanation (identified by the foul odor) dispersed in toilet air.[17] The issue of odor was also seen as an indicator of an inability to maintain cleanliness, which was largely associated with being uncivilized.[18] Meanwhile, in colonies, local people's lifestyle and sanitary behaviors were medicated as a pathology that caused them to be unable to maintain their own cleanliness.[19]

Such accounts of the practical and symbolic risks of miasmic air, however, would be compromised by night soil profit and a colonial context that adopted an economic way of approaching hygiene. The night soil tendering system, best adapted to satisfy the fiscal constraints of colonial governments, became a common practice in Asian colonies such as Shanghai and Hong Kong, financing public toilet services by night soil selling. In her study of pail public toilets provided by the colonial government in the Shanghai International Settlement from the 1860s, Huang argues that the high value of night soil in agriculture made the government compromise on profit and smell. Rather than deodorizing night soil, the government introduced different measures, such as fixing night soil removal hours and the close inspection of operations with the support of laws, to reduce the foul smell, helping sustain toilet services.[20]

In a similar manner, the Hong Kong colonial government treasured night soil value and tended night soil to the highest bidder. In a field that required public funds and land, the government was happy to operate the toilets on a quasi-commercial basis. This arrangement supported public toilet services while providing the government with night soil revenue. The costs of running a government toilet service had to be covered by selling night soil to contractors without incurring any increases in public expenditure. Night soil had great manurial value, which encouraged night soil contractors to offer a good price to collect it from toilets (both government-owned and privately owned), contributing to toilet cleanliness and urban hygiene. Indeed, the value of night soil was also a great incentive for private toilet operators to continue their services. The government encouraged Chinese business to enter the toilet market by giving concessions (e.g., low taxes) while reserving the power to oversee both government-owned and privately owned toilets. This required establishing order in urban hygiene through the regulation of toilet spatial reorganization and night soil removal practice, relieving the sanitation problem.

Therefore, the government resorted to coercion in the form of fines and disciplinary supervision, which, underpinned by law, dictated how Chinese were to use urban space and maintain toilet sanitation.[21] It is important to note what Philippa Levin comments about the instrumental function of law in colonies, she says that law was used to set a tone for civilizing the local society through upholding the moral premises of Christianity, furthermore implying colonial governments would not submit to the uncivilized local customs.[22] In doing so, a system of right (morality) was developed, and norms were set through the legislation of laws.[23] Morality was reflected in the form of self-discipline, which had its origin in Christian pastoral guidance, developed on the basis that guiding the people in accordance with the doctrine of God.[24] This specific disciplinary form guided people to true one's innermost truth; otherwise, the self would be dammed by God. Resting on the obligation of disciplining oneself, the local society was obliged to be subordinate to the government.

It was thus deemed necessary for the law to look to the Hong Kong colonial government's guidance in order to bring out the moralizing effects of public toilets, disciplining the behaviour of toilet users, operators and night soil contractors alike, inducing moral habits, so that the urban space might be used properly and achieve cleanliness. In the following, the effects on the colony's public toilet services will be examined from a political economy perspective (involving a quasi-commercial toilet operating mode) to better contextualize how surveillance and regulation of toilets was underpinned by law to ensure the sustainability of commercial toilet services offered by both the government and the Chinese business.

5.2.2 Close Surveillance: European Inspectors with the Help of Chinese Elites

To ensure that public toilet services were not carried out in a carte-blanche manner, the first regulation related to toilet operation was mainly concerned with night soil removal. Regulating removal was aimed at maintaining urban hygiene, as the typical removal practices generally caused street pollution in terms of physical mess or daytime odor. To this end, the *Ordinance for the Maintenance of Order and Cleanliness* was enacted when the public toilet system was introduced in 1867.[25] The ordinance is divided into two parts, one concerning dust bins and the other on night soil removal, and was specifically aimed at preventing noisome odor and other negative effects to the surrounding neighborhood; the latter is the focus of this section.

Removing night soil from government toilets was put under the sole charge of contractors who successfully tendered for yearly rights to do so. Considering the high value of night soil, contractors and privately owned toilet operators monitored the removal coolies' work to ensure that they did not steal any of the valuable commodities and supervised that the night soil was removed daily. In an effort to minimize any negative effects on the neighborhood through the course of removal, night soil was placed in buckets of uniform color and size with close fitting lids. The removal hours were fixed between midnight and seven or eight A.M., depending on the season. Furthermore, the conservancy boats were only allowed to berth at ten designated wharves between Saiyingpun and Causeway Bay. For any breach of the regulations, the contractors could be punished with a fine not exceeding HK$100 or imprisoned with or without hard labor for any period not exceeding three months.

In the early 1880s, a system of inspection was implemented to help enforce the regulations. This consisted of close surveillance of night soil removal and toilet conditions. Seeing the difficulties of maintaining urban hygiene and toilet cleanliness, as both government-owned and privately owned toilets were operated in a quasi-commercial mode through the selling of night soil, Chadwick strongly supported top-down oversight of night soil contractors and toilet operators in his report concerning the maintenance of general sanitation in 1882. He emphasized the importance of "the strongest necessity for inspection and supervision" by the government to ensure the sanitary condition of public toilets and that general sanitation was "provided with reasonable means for cleanliness" that would encourage the general Chinese public to carry out hygienic practices.[26] Based on Chadwick's suggestions, a series of government interventions aimed at ensuring that toilet services and night soil removal would not have ill effects on the surrounding neighbourhood was adopted in 1883, when the Sanitary Board was established.[27] The Surveyor General had been appointed by the governor to be the board chairman, who executed his duties with the assistance of the Colonial Surgeon and the Chinese Protector (or the Registrar General) who could speak Cantonese, under these appointments were the European inspectors and Chinese District Watchmen. To maintain urban hygiene, the government also regulated bodily behavior in public areas and the sanitary condition of public toilets in villages and gave responsibility for these to the police, who regularly checked the toilets to ensure they were properly lime washed once a month and were kept in a clean and inoffensive condition.[28]

This marked a new era of toilet administration in the colony, which is reflected in two aspects. First, this hierarchical surveillance system, consisting of watchmen at the lowest level, head watchmen and (senior) inspectors in the middle, and the Chinese Protector, Colonial Surgeon and Surveyor General at the top, was designed to closely surveil Chinese people to maintain urban hygiene. Such a system of surveillance was done practically by the inspectors, who enforced the sanitary codes from the Colonial Surgeon, and done politically by the watchmen from the Chinese Protector, who could speak Chinese and directed the general Chinese population through the watchmen's sanitary duties. Furthermore, from 1862, Chinese people were required to bring any petitions they had to the Protector, who would refer the petitions to the government on their behalf. So it seems that the Protector was their guide, and so they allowed him to exert discipline upon them.[29] Chinese were described by Chadwick as,

> A most docile people, and are accustomed for countless generations to implicit submission to authority. Once let them see that Government is in earnest about sanitation, and that whilst giving facilities, and interfering but little with their social custom, there is a firm determination to enforce cleanliness, there will be little or no resistance.[30]

Based on the notion of paternalism—putting colonial government and Chinese into a vertical framework of guardian and child—Chadwick paid special attention to the importance of the Protector in preserving hygiene, with the hope that the Protector would smooth any difficulties, for example, hostility towards government intervention into Chinese sanitary behaviors (e.g., improper bodily habits and maintaining toilet cleanliness), encountered by the inspectors during daily inspections. In doing so, the Protector could reduce resistance to sanitary measures while encouraging Chinese cooperation. This illustrated the colonial complexities that the Sanitary Board, consisting of not only medical and public health professionals but also an expert in Chinese culture, helped to smooth. In terms of regulating urban space, the government could not take its institutional capacity for granted when implementing public health policies, as the Chinese population was not simply an object that could be manipulated at will. As a number of scholars of colonialism, such as Arnold and Yeoh contend, sanitary measures were never enforced simply through coercion in the form of intrusive and hierarchical intervention or Western hegemony resting on the employment of public health knowledge. Rather, governments could only manage to implement their measures with the cooperation of the general community if it was to significantly sustain colonial rule.[31]

Second, to make the work of inspection more palpable to Chinese night soil contractors, toilet operators and users while reinforcing the European inspectors' work, the duty of enforcing urban hygiene was added to that of Chinese District Watchmen, who were included in the newly established Sanitary Board.[32] The policy included instructions for the supervisory role of the Inspector of Nuisances and Watchmen of daily night soil removal and toilet operation, helping to ensure toilet viability and the proper removal of night soil in populated places. The idea to recruit watchmen to enforce sanitary duties was suggested to Chadwick by Chinese elites in 1881, when he held meetings with influential Chinese social organizations such as TWH during his investigation of the colony's sanitary conditions.[33] The reason behind the suggestion is unclear, however, and whether elites consciously had a vested interest in supervising urban hygiene. One possibility might be upper class Chinese wanted to portray themselves as a governing power by positioning themselves as having superior morals concerning public interests, including public health, compared to their countrymen, such a move could reinforce their prestige and position as local leaders.[34] The vested interests appear to be consistent with the situation in other colonies, where local elites became increasingly concerned with sanitation to maintain property values or because of their own health concerns.[35] This meant they often had a shared interest and so worked with the colonizers in regulating urban hygiene towards the goal of enforcing control on their fellow countrymen.

Whatever the reason to suggest Chinese watchmen, the active role played by the homemade Chinese elites in urban governance reinforced vertical stratification within the Chinese community, the perception that there was a clear distinction between respectable and general Chinese. The crucial point is that the District Watchmen Force (DWF), set up and financed by homemade Chinese business elites in 1866, helped maintain a cultural hegemony over the general Chinese community, which was based on a long established Chinese hierarchical system, as noted in Chap. 2. As a political strategy, this allowed the government to involve the elites as strategic partners in the regulation of their fellow countrymen and urban space. The force was thoroughly Chinese in character, and watchmen posts were nominated by Chinese Kaifong (neighbor) leaders and appointed by the government. Eventually, the DWF was praised by Chadwick as an effective organization for enforcing sanitary rules.[36] Indeed, sanitary regulations could not simply be imposed by the government on the general Chinese population, and their enforcement required coordination with the elites, who financed the watchmen and supported them in supervising the sanitary requirements.

The cooptation of Chinese watchmen and government inspectors in maintaining urban hygiene was accompanied by a systematic policy of controlling night soil contractors and privately owned toilet operators. Each District Inspector of Nuisances (altogether three by 1883) had two head watchmen attached to him, and such watchmen carried out the instructions of the inspectors and reported to the inspectors their own observations of urban hygiene and those from their watchmen every day.[37] Nonetheless, both the inspectors and the head watchmen came under the supervision of a Senior Inspector of Nuisances, who inspected the night soil conservancy boats and public toilets on irregular days once a week, ensuring the inspectors and head watchmen were performing their duties efficiently and that the toilets were clean and orderly.[38] By the end of 1883, Victoria City was divided into six districts, each with three to eight watchmen led by a head watchman. In total, there were six head watchmen and 37 watchmen inspecting the night soil collection and public toilet system.[39] More practically, however, the watchmen looked for negligence or disobedience in following the instructions for night soil removal, as defined by the Sanitary Board. Except in cases of emergency, the inspectors did not give any instructions to the watchmen directly, mostly communicating to them through the head watchmen and holding the latter responsible for the actions and conduct of the watchmen. A special case is when a watchman apprehends an offender, who, for example, might have deposited night soil in a public area. In this case, the watchman should take the offender to the nearest police station, and conjointly with an inspector, charge the offender before a police magistrate. Part of the rationale for the arrangement to include only the removal of night soil and not the condition of the actual public toilets into the watchmen's duties might have been that removal was to be done following a set of standardized instructions (e.g., standardized night soil buckets and removal routes), and so was perceived by the government as an easier job for watchmen to supervise.

However, the involvement of watchmen in sanitary duties lasted only three years.[40] Hamilton alludes that perhaps Chinese business interests were reluctant to continue paying for watchmen, whose sanitary duties were larger than expected, or that business only participated in the first places because it was not strong enough to refuse the government when Chadwick first proposed the scheme to them.[41] The annual salary for head watchmen was HK$180, and for watchmen, it varied from HK$77 to HK$84. The salaries mainly drew from the District Watchman's Fund, which was financed by Chinese business. The government's annual subsidy was a mere HK$24 and HK$12 for each head watchman and watchman.[42] As Hamilton argues, the government appropriated the DWF for its own use, which transferred watchmen from the private domain to the public domain without incurring large additional expenses.[43] Originally, watchmen had been employed for a very specific purpose: to maintain law and order in the Chinese quarter to secure local business interests (more details in Chap. 2). What subsequently occurred is that the watchmen were put under the control of the government for sanitary duties, in equal importance to their other policing duties. The head watchmen having to report to the inspectors every day, putting them under the control of the inspectors, would have been regarded as "a loss of face" by the Chinese. Worse still, they were required to use their best endeavors to detect nuisances at all times and could be dismissed by the government if they were found to not actively cooperate in detecting poor behavior by night soil contractors or toilet operators.

The end of the watchmen involved in toiler issues might also partly stem from the long-held prejudice in the mind of the government that Chinese people were ignorant, regardless of their class, so the toilets should be put under the supervision of European inspectors. As Chadwick states clearly, these inspectors "could introduce habits of cleanliness to detect and remedy evils... operating under the personal direction of a responsible European officer".[44] This emphasized the policies of paternalism between Europeans and Chinese, underlining the assumption that Europeans had higher morality. For the government, it was absolutely necessary to appoint European inspectors who could better ensure that sanitary ordinances and instructions were followed. The surveillance of exercises relating to morality was expected to introduce morality to Chinese and help them understand that the government was a watchful one, which would render the colony healthier and more prosperous.[45] The inspectors were required to examine the toilets in their respective districts at least twice a week, ensuring that they were kept clean and odor free.[46] In the 1890s, this was made more frequent every morning, probably because of the high usage due to rapid population growth.[47] Furthermore, the duties became more specific, and they came to include ensuring that cleansing, disinfecting, lime-washing and tarring were conducted in toilets properly.

Nevertheless, inspectors could be bribed, or they may extort the toilet operators or toilet landowners, as shown in Chan Pui's case in Chap. 4. Furthermore, the inspectors could not speak Cantonese (one of the main dialects used in Hong Kong), causing problems in carrying out daily sanitary duties. Chinese interpreters were then hired to assist inspectors' daily inspections. Although the annual salary of the interpreters was a mere HK$180, the requirements for the post were rather high, meaning that the candidates had to go through an examination held by the Department of Surveyor General, which mainly consisted of viva translation from Chinese into English and vice versa. Translators needed the ability to communicate in Cantonese and Hakka—the two most common dialects in nineteenth-century Hong Kong—as well as basic arithmetic skills.[48] In contrast, the requirements to be an inspector were unclear, yet their annual salary was HK$720, fourfold that of interpreters.[49] Moreover, the inspector's remuneration included a housing allowance of HK$180 a year, a sedan chair hire allowance of HK$60 for five months during the hot season, and three uniform annually by 1883.[50]

5.2.3 A Self-Regulating System of Facility Management

Beyond the usual form of surveillance by inspectors and watchmen, there were other, nonhuman forms of surveillance also being used in public toilets. To generate the desired moral effects of toilets, the structure and material of the interior and facility were purposefully designed. As a colonial milieu (an ordered space and structure), both government-owned and privately owned toilets were configured by the government as a disciplining site that could be managed and observed. Following this logic, a system of visibility was implanted into toilet structures and spatial organization. The toilets had to be illuminated (oil or electricity) during their entire opening hours, from 5 A.M. to 10 P.M., to bring brightness and make the internal structure clearly visible.[51] This also meant that a normal state could be set through the employment of standardized principles, which made any deviation easy to identify. The divisions between toilet seats were required to be made of ferro-concrete slabs coated with white enamel, and the backs of the compartments lined with white-glazed tiles.[52] These measures not only enabled easy observation and surveillance of Chinese bodily behavior and toilet cleanliness but also embodied symbolic meanings of cleanliness (through white tiles and illumination), which were associated with good morality and order. As noted in Chap. 4, government toilets contained fewer seats (meaning fewer night soil buckets), but more public space in surrounding areas and ventilation facilities was required, as they did not benefit from spheres of influence. All these construction regulations meant higher costs. As in the case of the Chuk Hing Lane public toilet, considering the objections, the number of toilet seats was scaled down from 40 to 16, and the building was modified from two to one floor.[53]

To prevent dirt from accumulating, there was also particular concern given to the interior design and material of toilet facilities. To obtain the agreement of petitioners for the building of a public toilet on Wanchai Gap Road, the government took every precaution to prevent it from causing unpleasant smells or obscene sights.[54] For example, double airtight doors were provided, one of which had to be shut before the other was opened. Furthermore, much ventilation was installed to improve air circulation. Instead of simple ventilation that consisted only of diffusion through windows and electric exhaust fans (HK$30 per month was budgeted for running it), there was an elaborate system of controlled ventilation by means of an upright shaft that was fixed above the highest point in the roof, ensuring foul air ascended to the highest point. Moreover, cremating furnaces for the foul air were provided at the outlets before the air passed outside. The importance of installing fans to preserve the manurial value of the night soil is clearly shown in a report related to toilet cleanliness published in 1899. The report reflects how the innovations in toilet construction and management were aimed at preserving the value of the night soil while minimizing the odor. The Sanitary Surveyor, R. F. Drury, explained that,

> Owing to the large amount of ventilation that will be provided I do not recommend lessening the value of the manure and doubling the quantity to be handled by admixture with red earth but continuing as hitherto, leaving it plain with a good provision of disinfectants about the latrine.[55]

Similar fears about dirt accumulation and odor are also found in Chadwick's report, where he suggests there should be no sharp or hidden corners or spaces in which dirt could become lodged, as these would be more difficult to routinely clean.[56] The above specifications relating to toilet interiors and facility building materials in the colony were applied consistently, similar to the view of sanitarians in the West that believed a self-regulating system of facility management could keep toilets in order, helping to ensure cleanliness. For example, smooth and non-absorbent materials were used while the use of wood was avoided. Internal walls were paved with white-glazed polished tiles, and floors were cemented, tiled, or covered with asphalt, as mentioned. Granite was avoided because its rough surface easily retained dirt and moisture. Meanwhile, night soil buckets and footrests were made of corrugated iron to prevent oxidization, and reinforced concrete, brick or glazed tiles that would not easily absorb dirt; boat-shaped night soil buckets made of earthenware or zinc were substituted for wooden buckets, enabling the facilities to be kept clean.[57] Nonhuman surveillance occurred as an indirect inspection by making the interior design and building materials of toilets conform to the same specifications (regulatory standards), helping to impose the same regulations on every night soil contractor and toilet operator.

More disciplined behavior on the part of night soil contractors and toilet operators was regarded as important to improving toilet cleanliness. Such behavior was legally regulated from 1885 for government toilets and 1891 for privately owned ones.[58] This legal framework made contractors and operators liable to prosecution if a government or privately owned toilet was found to be in a bad state. The implementation of these new regulations may reflect insufficient human or nonhuman surveillance in maintaining toilet cleanliness, thus requiring the passage of laws that introduce clearer standards of compliance that hold contractors and operators legally responsible. For example, an able-bodied adult toilet attendant was required to be made present, and the attendant should constantly be on duty. They needed to lime wash the interior walls, tar any fittings made of wood at least once every lunar month, and thoroughly scrub all channels, floors, partitions, seats, and utensils at least once every day with detergent and deodorant. Furthermore, the contents of night soil buckets were covered with dry earth, opium packing, or saw dust, and fumigants were burned during opening hours. Such practices were enforced in government toilets in 1885, and then they were suddenly put in force in private toilets in 1891, at the beginning of a boom in the commercial public toilet industry.[59]

5.2.4 Intervention in Disease Outbreaks

Tension between the government and business persisted, especially when the government disposed of or disinfected night soil from government public toilets during epidemics.[60] The night soil contractor who successfully bid for the rights to the night soil collected in government public toilets could claim compensation for any loss that may have resulted from such disposal or disinfection. However, the government had no power to order private toilets to disinfect their night soil; it could only fine toilet operators who refused to disinfect their night soil during an epidemic.

Disinfection orders were first carried out after the 1894 plague.[61] The justification was that public toilets, particularly private toilets, were seen to be a major source and medium of transmission of the plague. In a medical report, *The Epidemic of Bubonic Plague in Hong Kong, 1894*, the acting superintendent of Government Civil Hospital, J. A. Lowson, announced that "one of the most important factors in the spread of the disease was the bad condition of the latrines".[62] The evidence was that plague bacteria were abundant in public toilet night soil. It was believed there was a correlation between disease, night soil itself and the gas it generated. This miasmatic theory argued that disease is caused and spread by an air-born substance, described as a gas, that emanates from various solids, such as an animal, carcass or fecal matter. (Description of miasma theory.) The public health implication of the theory is that disease and infection can occur not just from direct contact with fecal matter but also through the inhalation of the gas. Supporting this theory was that poor Chinese men, who frequently visited or lived near the toilets, appeared to be the most susceptible to the plague. A large number of deaths were found in houses around the toilets at 50 Center Street (owned by Kwok Acheong's family), 256 Queen's Road West (Tang Luk's family) and 82 First Street (Hu Tso). Regarding the high deaths recorded in Sheung Fung Lane, Lowson emphasized that "the inhabitants were principally night-soil coolies and *almost all died* (italics original)."[63] There were two public toilets near Sheung Fung Lane: one at 91 s Street and the other at 113 s Street. In light of this, some immediate measures, such as temporarily closing any surrounding houses that had more than three deaths.

The 1894 plague killed 2,485 people, approximately one percent of the total population, including military garrisons (estimated population was 246,006 by December 1894).[64] As a result, compradors, tradesman and even coolies fled Hong Kong; in total, approximately 100,000 people and nearly all Chinese shops were closed, even though the large sugar refineries stopped operating.[65] Clearly, the plague was a serious issue for commercial and government revenue. A second outbreak eventually compelled the government to enforce more stringent sanitary measures for maintaining toilet cleanliness, including dispatching garrisons to assist sanitary inspectors. There was also a drive to disinfect night soil in public toilets, and disinfection became so important that 10,000 lbs of chlorinated lime was used in 1895 alone.[66] There was some reluctance on the part of privately owned toilet operators to comply with the order; the operators of the facilities in Gough Street and Heung Lane were therefore subject to legal proceedings and fined HK$25 and HK$50 by the magistrate. However, these toilets continued to provide services after the plague without many operational changes, which is reflected in the continued complaints regarding their poor cleanliness and condition.[67] Seeing this and noting that there was no incentive for landowners to provide domestic toilets in dwellings, Lowson called for the introduction of public toilets throughout Victoria City to be maintained exclusively by the government to a good standard. However, the call was not heeded, and under consideration of fiscal constraints and the threat to land revenue, no prompt action was taken.

5.2.5 *Effectiveness of Regulations*

In response to the poor standard of privately owned toilets, an injunction system was established by the Supreme Court. Ultimately, however, this was ineffective at stopping the construction of new public toilets. For example, is the case of Pang Tai Yuen and Kwong Kam Tong. The two men entered into a partnership to build a private toilet at 23 West Street in 1893.[68] However, they were strongly challenged. Lee Ching, who owned two nearby properties, spoke against the new facility and asked for a perpetual injunction to restrain a public toilet from being built on the property or in any other place that would depreciate the value of her properties.[69] Lee and several residents from the neighborhood provided evidence for the alleged nuisance and depreciation of property value in court. It was established that there was a potential nuisance, and the court granted an injunction.[70] However, the injunction was short-lived, and Pang eventually established a toilet at the site two years later in 1895 (refer to Table 4.6).

Even with the injunction power of the courts, it is evident that such instances of even a temporary stoppage to a public toilet were uncommon. Despite continuous complaints from landowners near Chan Pui's toilet at 2 Gough Street since its opening in 1891, his toilet was allowed to operate until the 1920s (Table 4.6). The most serious complaint against Chan was perhaps a court case made by Ng Tat Chi in 1896, where Ng claimed that the gases from the ventilators of Chan's toilet entered his home at 12 Aberdeen Street, diagonally opposite the toilet building.[71] Ng applied for an injunction in the Supreme Court and aimed to recover HK$100 damages to cause discomfort. The Court fined Chan a reduced HK$20 but declined the injunction, owing to insufficient public toilets in the area and because Chan showed interest in continuing the toilet business. However, the government considered closing Chan's toilet as early as 1904,[72] when a miasma nuisance was claimed to have caused sickness among teachers of Belilios Public School next to the toilet building. However, the court decided to take no action when it found that nearby inhabitants greatly needed access to the public toilet. For Chan's toilet, it was the only toilet in the vicinity, and the facility unfortunately needed to stay open. It would appear Chan had a local monopoly on the toilet market, and the infrastructure was too critical to close regardless of the harms.

These public nuisance issues caused by night soil might have been the result of a compromise between night soil profit and toilet cleanliness: the economic sustainability of the limited privately owned public toilet network was critical, as the population was growing and government public toilets and domestic toilet services were inadequate. The high demand for toilet services allowed privately owned public toilet operators and owners to advance their own interest. It is worth noting that the government did support these toilets, creating the conditions in which the business sector was required to participate to maintain the most basic sanitation coverage. On the one hand, the government protected toilet profits while securing the ongoing operation of privately owned public toilets through its legal apparatus. For example, the court proceedings and the enactment of a Bye law on public toilets in 1890 that restricted competitors' entry into the toilet market secured the interests of existing toilet owners, encouraging them to continue toilet services. On the other hand, it maintained general toilet cleanliness by imposing fines, monitoring facilities closely and employing technologies, such as powerful air-jet systems to exhaust foul air.

However, the introduction of new, regulating legislation did not always bring the expected results. The ordinances and supervision system pertaining to the management of toilets and night soil removal were sometimes neither abided by nor strictly enforced. Fines against operators that failed to keep their public toilets in the correct condition were laid infrequently. For example, during the period of 1885–1905, which includes the decades before and after the 1894 plague, no prosecutions were registered in 1885, 1889 to 1893, 1896, and 1897. There were only four fines in the year of the plague, 1894, and the year with the most fines was 1903, when 23 fines were issued, but only for a total amount of HK$239.[73] Acting to maximize their profit, toilet operators paid little attention to potential fines, so no further steps to improve the toilet condition appear to have been taken. This is reflected in the poor toilet conditions documented at the end of the nineteenth century.[74] In the meantime, the government did not strictly enforce the provision with public funds or land, as it understood that the limited nature of the existing toilet services was a state in fact favored by Chinese business. Hence, enforcement of sanitary measures was depreciated in every possible way.

Nonetheless, the toilet market was created and further sharpened through successive rounds of regulation. By examining the regulation and surveillance of daily toilet practices, this section illustrates how the government *used political techniques (the employment of District* Watchmen and a hierarchical *inspection system) to* diminish the negative effects of night soil on the public. Sanitary measures specifically aimed to discipline night soil contractors and toilet operators to create sanitary toilet conditions, which was important to introduce public health discourses to lower-class Chinese toilet users. Furthermore, the government decided to deodorize and disinfect toilets, rather than night soil, which was a compromise between urban regulation and night soil profit. Such efforts also largely reduced the requirement for night soil deodorization and disinfection, which would have lessened the value of the night soil. Through maintaining the profitability of the toilets, their viability and contribution to general sanitation were secured.

The government's effort to shape a toilet market that was profitable and moral also created a capitalist class that was integral to the colony's functioning. Those Chinese businesses who were able to become established in the toilet market became an institutional part of the colony's governance, public service provision and economy. Indeed, the actual construction of such urban order was never a straightforward, top-down exercise; instead, it was always enabled by multiple sources of power, such as the district watchmen, European inspectors and the Chinese Protector (furthermore, we will see the role of toilet landowners and other elites in the next section), that traversed racial boundaries and the public and private spheres. Therefore, we need to consider the specific situation of early colonial Hong Kong, including the economic development and land power of Chinese elites, that came to act on the political (moral governance on general Chinese and toilet cleanliness) and economic sustainability of the toilets. Indeed, the bulk of public toilet facilities were provided by business interests and were the product of both regulation and profit accumulation of urban space. Therefore, the sustainability of toilets cannot be separated from the economic strategies of the elites.

5.3 Chinese Business: Land Resources and Social Networks

As seen earlier, the most difficult aspect for the government in establishing new public toilets was finding appropriate land to do so. Toilets needed to be near population centers, but as the facility could damage nearby property values, the government needed to negotiate with the powerful landowners, which often led to abandoning potential toilet sites. In contrast, the self-interest of toilet landowners encouraged them to contain the negative aspects of a public toilet facility, namely, the noisome odor, and so they were able to successfully sustain toilet services, despite the inefficiencies. The sustainability of any particular public toilet facility can be defined with two indicators: first, long-term operation at the same address (Table 4.6), and second, being free of public complaints. This certainly does not mean that privately owned toilets received no complaints, as noted earlier, but the number was much fewer compared to government ones, and the complaints were not made by powerful landowners but simply nearby residents.

The difference in complaints suggests that the control of land and social networks was the key factor for toilet landowners to ensure the long-term sustainability of their toilets. They made use of two interacting resources: land and social networks. It was a combination of great amounts of land belonging to the same toilet landowners, who formed buffers around their toilets to minimize complaints, and the interlocking relationships (such as relatives or friends) between toilet landowners and other elites, that made the latter willing to accept these toilets in the vicinity of their properties. The following will show how burgeoning power, derived from extensive land holdings, enabled toilet landowners to employ economic strategies in the enforcement of the public pail toilet system.

5.3.1 The Spheres of Influence

The extensive involvement of Chinese landowners in the public toilet market after the late 1860s significantly transformed the urban landscape. Toilets from this time, located in the circular pathway, Des Voeux Road Central, Heung Hing Lane, Pound Lane, Queen's Road West and Sam To Lane, all stood in the same locations for many years, as noted in Chap. 4. Some toilets were located at the end of narrow lanes to hide them from public noses and eyes to minimize the negative effects of the toilet on the neighbourhood. Clearly, the landowners understood that the nature of the public toilets could be a serious public nuisance in a densely populated urban space. The most important concern, however, was to sustain toilet services and secure toilet gains. In this vein, toilet landowners exercised their land power and resources by establishing privately owned toilets in locations surrounded by properties that they owned, which operated as a 'sphere of influence'. Economically, this addressed the potential for complaints due to the foul odor emanating from public toilets, a serious issue in the densely populated Chinese quarter. This helped to keep toilet services running and solved the problem faced by the government in how to manage the daily needs of lower-class Chinese and maintain urban hygiene.

The development of the sphere is elaborated below. Even in the initial period of building a privately owned toilet, most toilets were strategically built adjacent to properties that belonged to the same toilet landowner, reflecting an intention to control any spillover consequences of the noisome air that may affect the lives of nearby residents. It must be noted, however, that it is not that property investment became centered around toilet services but rather that opportunistic investment developed a peculiar situation that involved forming spheres of influence. To attract the most business, privately owned toilets were often situated in very busy locations, where considerable amounts of night soil and entry fees could be collected. Land in these locations was worthy of investment, attracting landowners who had a strong market sense.

The development process of the spheres is marked by two stages: first, the mid-1860s to mid-1870s; and second, the late-1870s to late-1890s. Each phase is closely related to the amount of land that was controlled by toilet landowners. Seeing the vibrant land market, wealthy Chinese fleeing to Hong Kong due to the Taiping Rebellion from the early 1860s hastened to invest in the local property market. Nevertheless, they became much more heavily involved in the land market under the administration of Governor Hennessy from the late 1870s onwards. This is reflected in their tax paid, which was mainly based on land investment. In the early twentieth century, however, fluctuating silk and night soil demand, due to the combined effects of natural disasters and political turmoil in Guangdong Province, meant that landowners withdrew from the toilet market, and therefore the spheres were dismantled.

In the first stage, the spheres were formed in a piecemeal manner: toilets were installed adjacent to a single or a few of the toilet landowner's properties, which became a buffer; however, soon more properties were added, all owned by the same toilet landowner. The zones gradually grew as more properties adjoining the toilet facilities were added, and then larger coverage areas comprising whole neighborhoods, and then a 'sphere of influence'. However, the boundaries of such spheres were not clearly defined. There are two main patterns in the spatial arrangement of the sphere. First, a street-side toilet may be situated in between two properties owned by the toilet landowner. Second, the toilet facility may be located on a street corner, with the toilet landowner's properties on either side. For example, Chung Lo Luey (the owner of the Pond Street public toilet), Kwok Acheong (First Street and Pound Lane), Lee A Lok (Heung Hing Lane), Loo Yew Urh (Pond Lane), How A Shun (Mercer Street), Ng Sang (Rutter Lane), and Wong A Shing (Eastern Street) all arranged their spheres in this pattern.[75] It is unclear whether Wong was also Wong Shing the Legislative Councilor, who was father-in-law to a prominent Chinese leader, Wei Yuk. These three patterns were present for a decade until the mid-1870s, when more Chinese landowners emerged, which led to a drastic change in the public toilet landscape.

As more land came under the control of toilet landowners, they were inevitably able to strengthen their spheres of influence. During the second stage of sphere

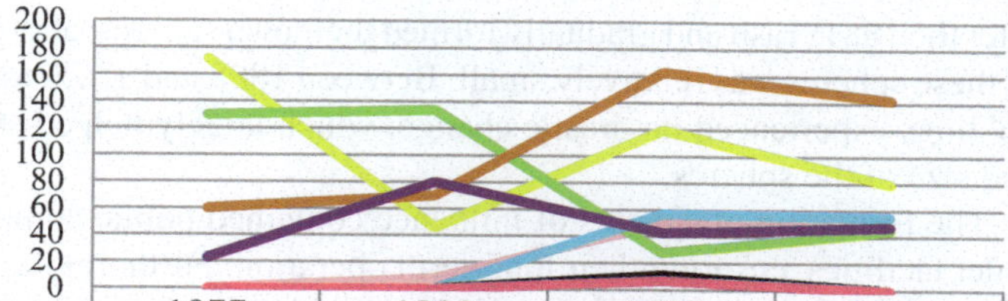

	1877	1880	1888	1895
Choy Chan	172	46	120	80
Ip Ching Chuen	0	8	50	55
Kwok A Cheong	130	134	28	45
Ng Ping Sam	0	0	57	55
Pow Ping Kwan	0	0	11	0
Tang Luk	60	70	163	143
Tso Wing Yung	23	80	43	48
Tsui Cheong lung	0	0	7	0
Total	385 (0)	338 (4)	478 (8)	434(7)

Fig. 5.1 Landownership of main toilet landowners in Victoria City, 1877–95 (pieces of land). *Source* The author compiled and computed the figures based on the names of the toilet landowners and their family members from HKRS38-2-23, 38-2-33, 38-2-57, 38-2-81, *RB*, 1877, 1880, 1888, 1895

formation from the late 1870s to late 1890s, the number of spheres increased significantly: four (1880), eight (1888) and seven (1895) spheres were formed in west Victoria City (Fig. 5.1). One point to be noted here is that the number and size of the spheres was closely associated with the land investment of the toilet landowners. A rough calculation of land ownership and purchases in 1877, 1880, 1888 and 1895 finds that eight toilet landowners held at least 385, 338, 487 and 471 land parcels in west Victoria City, respectively (Fig. 5.1). It is possible to trace the development and changing location of their land holdings. Four large toilet landowners (Choy Tang, Kwok Acheong, Tang Luk, and Tso Wing Yung) began to purchase more land in the late 1870s, and soon afterwards, they entered the toilet market.

Like many others, toilet landowners were highly involved in land price speculation, so the size of their land holdings greatly fluctuated. Kwok's and Tso's spheres shrank after the 1881 property crush, in which a large number of Chinese landowners suffered huge losses.[76] The number and size of spheres belonging to Kwok and Tso decreased in parallel with a reduction in their overall land holdings, from 134 to 28 and 80 to 43 properties from 1881 to 1888. Kwok Acheong died in 1880, and his sons suffered great property losses in the property crash, subsequently going into financial difficulty. From 1882, they faced a series of court cases, and Kwok Hew Kai declared bankruptcy in 1883.[77] While their spheres decreased, other toilet landowners, such as Choy Chan and Tang Luk, bought land to increase the number and size of their own spheres. Furthermore, Ip Ching Chuen and Ng Ping Sam began to buy more land after the 1881 crash and gradually formed their own spheres, although the overall size of these spheres was relatively small. Between 1888 and 1895, toilet landowner land holdings experienced no drastic change, which largely helped stabilize the number and size of the spheres.

The formation of spheres of influence contained public complaints about public toilet facilities, ensuring their long-term operation. Furthermore, without needing to be concerned about nearby complaints, toilet landowners did not need to deodorize the air, disinfect the night soil, or burn fumigants in the toilets. There was no need to invest too much in toilet cleanliness, allowing landowners to generate more profits by reducing operating costs. Being able to minimize operating costs was certainly an incentive for landowners to continue toilet services. Through toilet owner control of land resources, the sustainability of privately owned toilets was guaranteed as long as properties in the vicinity were controlled by the same toilet landowner and could successfully be passed to the next generation. For example, the toilets at 38 circular pathways (owned by Tang Luk), 116 Des Voeux Road Central (Choy Chan) and 3 Sam To Lane (Ip Ching Chuen) survived for two or three generations for over seven decades (refer to Table 4.6).

The formation of spheres was an economic strategy that drew upon these landowners' advantageous structural position in the hierarchy of land hegemony. In other words, the sustainability of privately owned toilets was closely linked to toilet landowner family wealth, which was based on land investment. It was their peculiar capacity as major landowners that enabled them to exercise that land power. In doing so, they not only helped commit land to public services, saving crown land and funds but also addressed the potential for complaints, and so made a mass pail public toilet system sustainable (Fig. 5.2).

5.3.2 *Web of Relationships and Reciprocal Obligations*

The successful operation of spheres of influence was not solely dependent on strategic land investment but was also based upon numerous relationships between toilet landowners and other elites. These relationships facilitated the exchange of reciprocal obligations, increasing the returns of cooperation. Axelrod argues that the pursuit of self-interest encourages cooperation because of reciprocity. He suggests that some conditions, such as the durability and frequency of interaction, affect and strengthen the terms of relationships among the players. As such, there are then expectations for future gains in continued contacts, which induce reciprocal obligations, and such obligations make each party consider one another when making decisions and incentives for cooperation.[78] Therefore, cooperation is more likely amongst people coming from a small area and members of social organizations or groups of acquaintances in which people would see each other on a regular basis.

In practice, the unique political-economic situation in the early colonial years was particularly encouraging for cooperation among Chinese elites. The number of elites was quite small, and therefore, it is not surprising that there were many

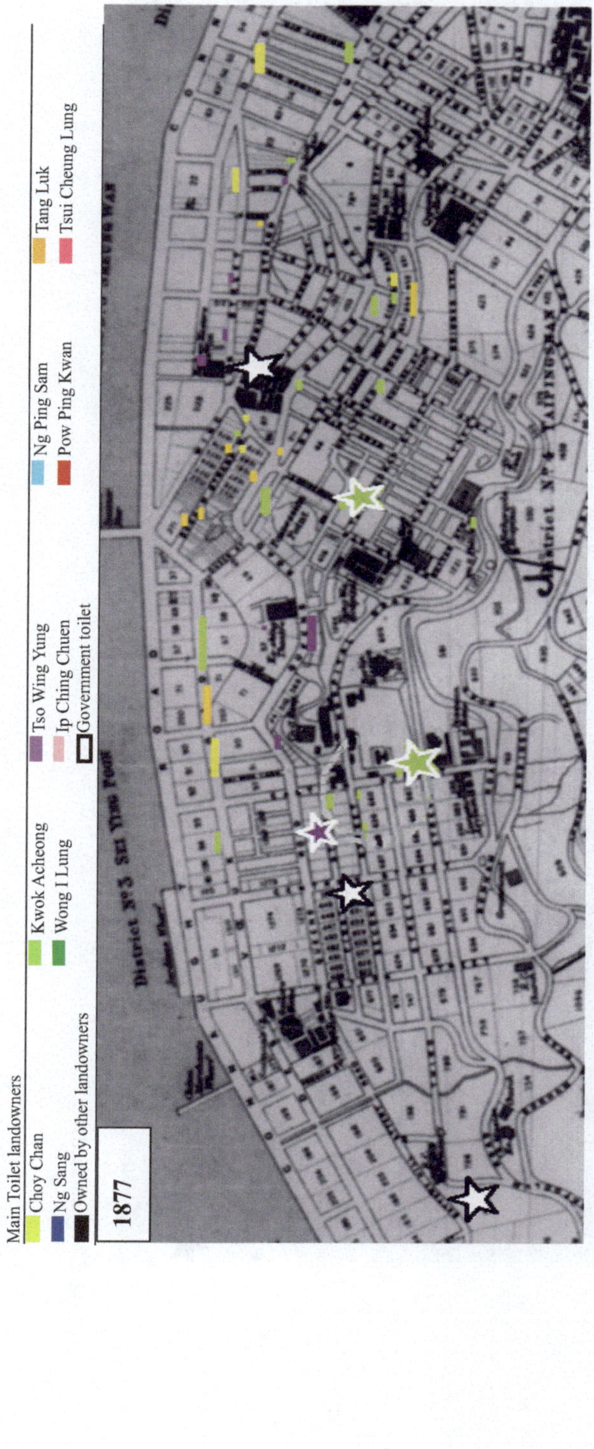

Fig. 5.2 Spheres of influence in West Victoria City, 1870s–1890s

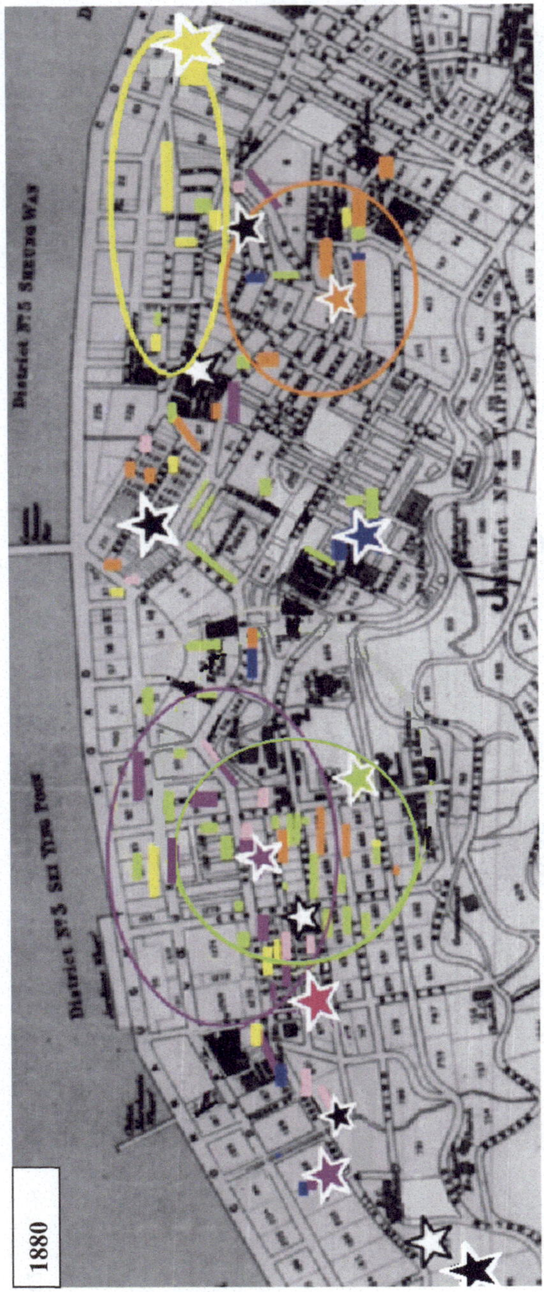

Fig. 5.2 (continued)

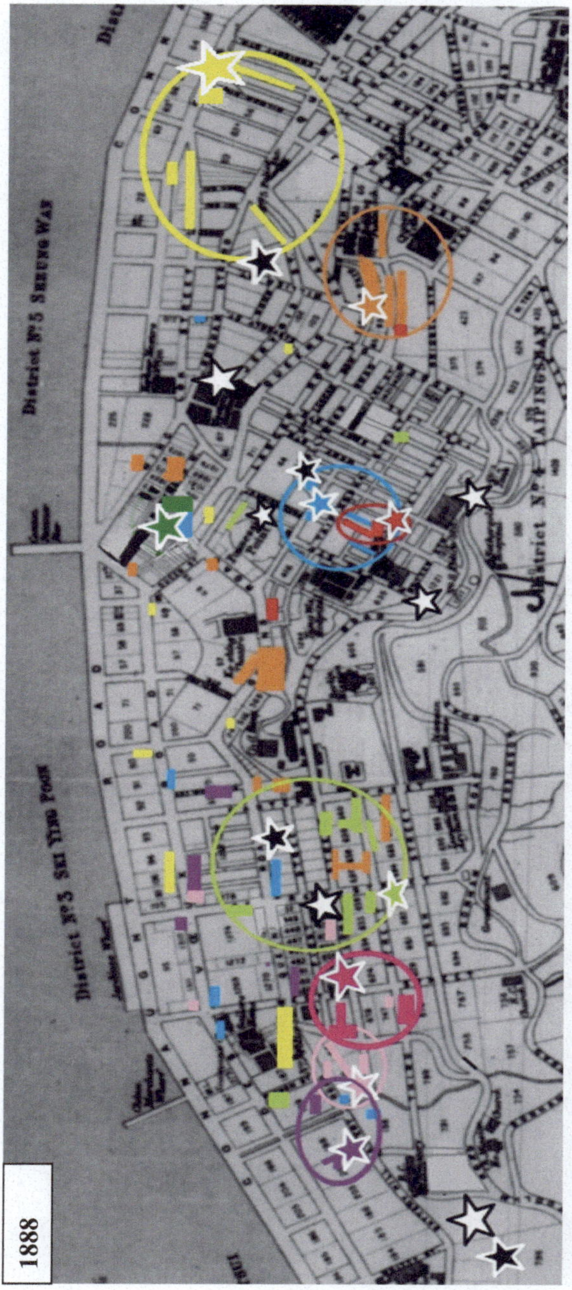

Fig. 5.2 (continued)

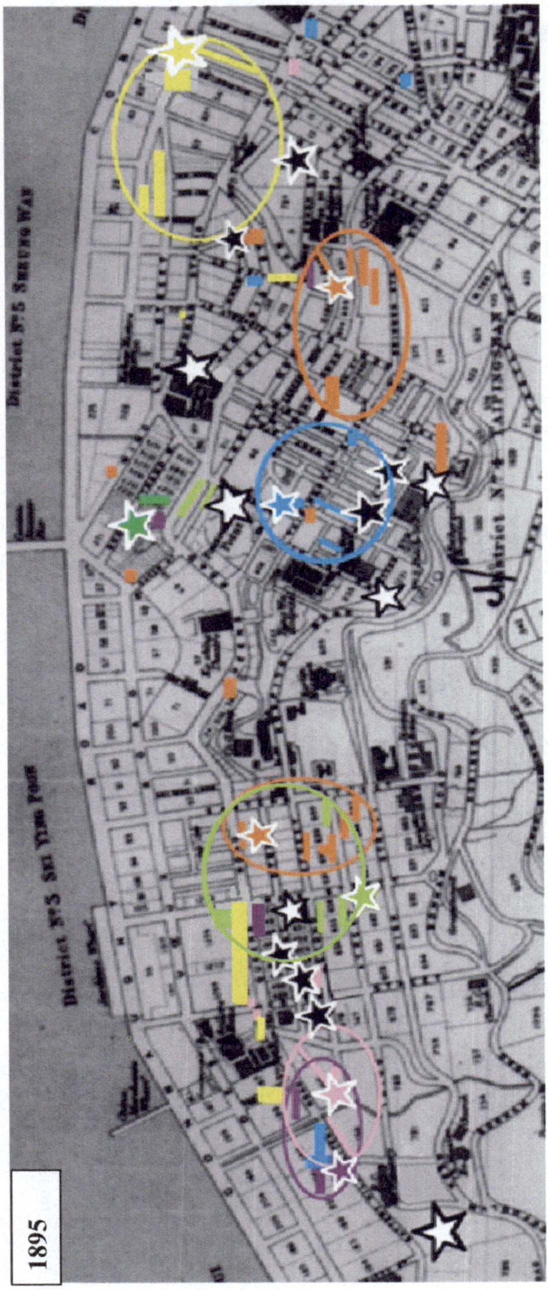

Fig. 5.2 (continued)

interlocking relationships between them.[79] For example, Chan's study of fourteen nineteenth-century Chinese Legislative Councilors notes that "nine of them were close kins of at least one other member among the fourteen... It is possible that if more distant kinship ties were included, *they might turn out to be just one big family* (italics added)".[80] Such interlocking relationships are also found among toilet landowners and other elites. They might be trading partners, members of the same social organizations (TWH or PLK) or government consultation committees, so there were many meetings and social events that took place that increased the frequency of regular interaction. This certainly made it easier to develop cooperative relationships and, on the basis of reciprocity or frequent interaction in socioeconomic fields, served as a strong incentive to not complain about public toilet nuisances on one's tenants or property.

Operating a sphere successfully required the collective effort of toilet landowners and their landowner friends. The entangled ties (personal, social, business, and political) bound toilet landowners and other elites together in multilevel networks, meaning they would respect each other's interests while pursuing their own. This allowed them to provide toilets more effectively than the government, most notably in terms of being able to offer toilet services at the same site for long periods of time. Unsurprisingly, some privately owned toilets adjoined other powerful landowners' or elites' land; however, complaints were seldom made about toilets that were owned or operated on by friends or relatives. Even with just a brief look at the *Rate Book* for the period around the late nineteenth century, it is clear that the majority of land in Victoria City was controlled by many of the toilet landowners' friends or relatives, such as Ho Tsoi, Ho Tung, Ip Chuk Kai, Jardine Matheson, Tsang Koon Man, and Wo Hang Opium Firm, which was owned by a partnership of Li Sing and Li Tak Cheong.[81] As a "friend" of the toilet owner, an obligation to not complain about a toilet facility could be developed.

The connections between toilet landowners and other elites, especially Chinese, existed in four layers: close and extended family, personal friends, business partners, and social connections (Fig. 5.3, also make reference to Table 5.1). An analysis of the multilayered relationships indicates that there existed a very tight network among them. While operating as a platform for the Chinese elites to provide social services to lower class Chinese, the Chinese social organizations, such as PLK and TWH, also allowed elites to establish closer relationships among the upper echelons of Chinese political and economic power in Hong Kong. The familial ties between toilet landowners and other elites were close. The best example to illustrate these interlocking relationships is marriage, which was used as a strategic instrument to strengthen family status and wealth. In studying Austrian Habsburg dynastic marriages in the sixteenth century, Fichtner notes that the pattern of strategic marriages among the ruling class was more frequent when people moved into the class, which indicates that "marriage policies were shaped by considerations other than those of simple preferential association within a select group".[82] "Dynastic strategy" is the term used by Fichtner to define these marriage arrangements, and the success of this strategy was made possible by targeting a suitable match. In his

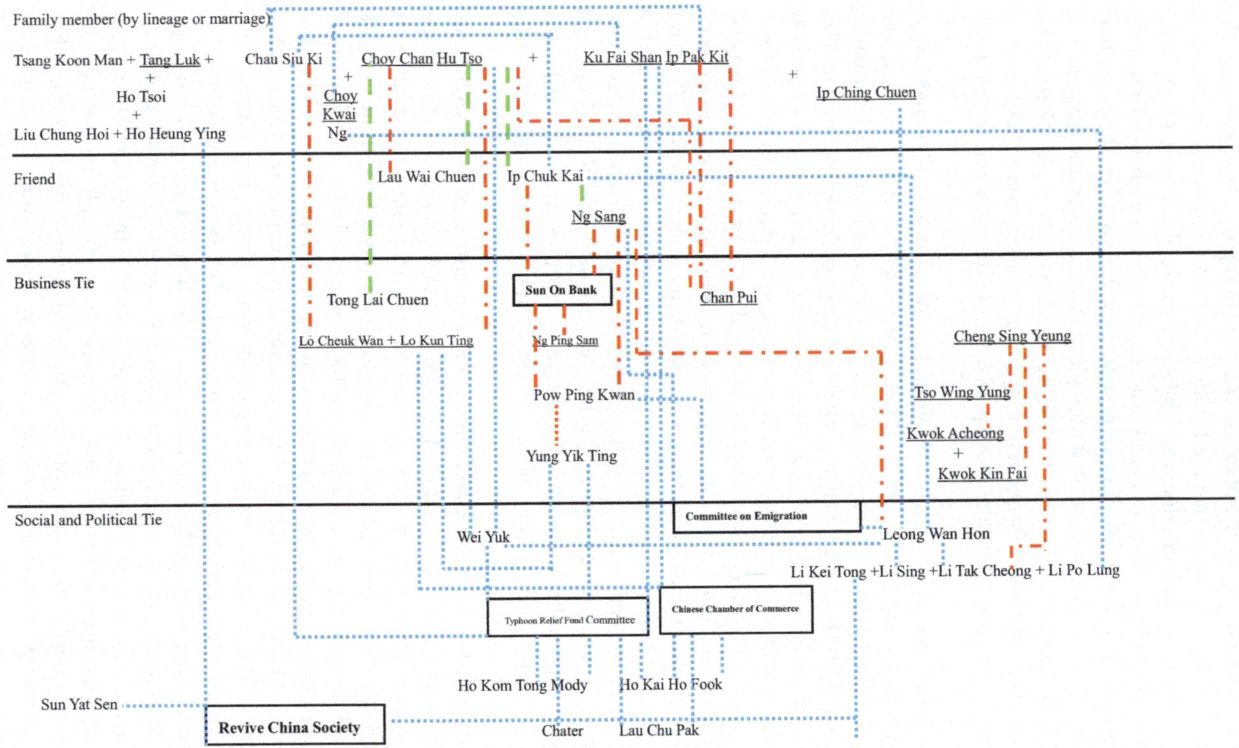

Fig. 5.3 Web of relationship between toilet landowners and other elites. *Source* Author research based on the following sources: Carl Smith Collection; *GG*, 1865–1920; PLK Archive; TWH Archive. *Note* (1) Bold letter stands for toilet landowner; +Family member; – – Friend; · – Business tie; ······ Social tie. (2) Due to limited coverage, the figure does not show all relationships between them

Table 5.1 Main toilet-landowners' profile

Name	Other business or occupation	Organization membership	Political appointment
Chan Pui	• Monopoly of slaughtering cattle • Night soil contractor • Scavenging contractor		
Cheong Assow	• Cattle dealer • Measurer of Land in Surveyor General Department • Overseer of coolies		
Cheng Sing Yeung	Tak On Bank founder	Member of Hong Kong General Chamber of Commerce	
Choy Kwai Ng	Shewan and Tomes & Co. comprador	• PLK: 1905/06 • TWH: 1906/07	
Hu Tso	• Cheong Fat Ferry Co. director • Government Civil and Lock Hospitals supplier • Imperial Bank of China shareholder • Kwong Wai Opium Farm partner • Monopoly of Slaughtering Cattle • Scavenging contractor	PLK: 1894/95, 1897/98	JP: 1902–05
Ip Ching Chuen	Hong Kong, Canton and Macao Steamboat Co	PLK: 1881/82	
Ku Fai Shan	• Po Lung Firm managing director • Shun On Steamship Co. partner • Tai Yau Opium Firm partner	• Founding member of Chinese Chamber of Commerce • PLK: 1894/95, 1901/02, 1905/06 • TW: 1895/96	Typhoon Relief Fund Committee
Kwok Acheong	• Bakery • Cosmopolitan Dock Co. director and shareholder • Fat Hing Firm founder • Monopoly of Slaughtering Cattle • Peninsular and Oriental Steam Navigator Co. comprador	• Kai Fong Committee member • PLK: Initiator • TWH: founding member and director-1873/74, 1879/80	
Lo Kun Ting	• Cheong Fat Ferry Co. director • China Merchants Steam Navigation Co. general manager • Dealer in Japanese good and opium • Kwong Wing Shang Lacquer proprietor • Tung On Fire Insurance director	• Founding member of Chinese Chamber of Commerce • PLK: 1897/98, 1899/1900 • TWH: 1899/1900	

(continued)

Table 5.1 (continued)

Name	Other business or occupation	Organization membership	Political appointment
Ng Sang	• Douglas Lapraik & Co. comprador • Wong Li Cheng Hong partner		Committee on Emigration of Women to the United States
Ng Ping Sam	Sun On Bank banker		
Pang Wa	• Tung Fung Chan rice store • Yick Sau Tong herbal shop		
Pow Ping Kwan	• Chinese Insurance Company partner • Olyphant & Co. comprador • Sun On Bank banker	TW: 1874/75, 1878/79, 1883/84	Committee on Emigration of Women to the United States
Tang Luk	Yuen Cheong Hong (stone quarrying)		
Wong I Lung	Monopoly of Slaughtering Cattle		

Source The author compiled the information from the following sources: Carl Smith Collection; PLK Archive; TWH Archive

opinion, marriage set the rules that governed the relationship and established obligations among family groups. Intermarriage between high-status families is particularly valuable, as it can prime each family for reciprocal exchange and thus can lead to enormous expansions of power.

Toilet landowners participated in the use of family to build political capital. One example is Hu Tso's daughter, who married Ku Fai Shan's son[83]; both fathers were newly rising Chinese elites, and Directors of PLK in 1894/5 will show later. Above all, however, the family of Tang Luk was the most complex. When Tang successfully moved into the ranks of the Chinese elite, he negotiated with another new elite, Tsang Koon Man, a stone quarry contractor and landowner, in the marriage between his third son, Tang Wing Tai, and Tsang's elder daughter, Tsang Jo Kiu.[84] Like Tang, Tsang was also a famous and wealthy stone quarry contractor and builder, and he later became a director of PLK (1885/6).[85] Tsang was also the founder of Tsang Tai Uk, the walled Hakka big house in today's Shatin, New Territories. He left an estate of HK$20,000 and huge land holdings in Shaukeiwan on Eastern Hong Kong Island in 1888.[86]

The same arrangement was repeated with Tang Luk's grandson (Tang Wing Tai's son), Tang Yung Mau, and Chau Lai Wah, the daughter of Chau Siu Ki, renowned as a

JP, Legislative Councilor, Tai Sun Bank managing partner, and real estate developer (manager of Hong Kong and Kowloon Land and Loan Co. in the early twentieth century).[87] Tang Luk's great grandson (Tang Yung Mau's son), Tang Man Chiu, married Ho Chit Shu (granddaughter of Ho Tsoi) in 1927. Ho Tsoi was naturalized as a British subject in 1899, and he was a large landowner and trader. He owned Cheung Fat Shang, a medicine shop, and Tseung On, a famous tea trading enterprise.[88] Ho's other granddaughter, Ho Chor Therefore, was the daughter-in-law of Tang King Po, a leading industrialist in the mid-twentieth century. His ninth daughter, Ho Heung Ying, was a member of the revolutionary Revive China Society, set up by Sun Yat Sen, the national father of China, in Hawaii. She and her husband, Liu Chung Hoi, and Li Kei Tong, the son of tycoon Li Sing, were all followers of Sun.[89]

It is worth noting that the toilet landowners also had many interlocking business connections. As shown in the previous chapter, Hu Tso sold his toilet on First Street to Lo Kun Ting. Hu's other toilet on Queen's Road West was originally established by Kwok in 1868 and was later run in a partnership with Tso Wing Yung before being transferred to the latter in 1873 (refer to Chap. 4). Meanwhile, a partnership was formed between Chan Pui and Ku Fai Shan over the Mercer Street privately owned public toilet, as shown earlier. Furthermore, toilet landowners commonly established positive business relationships with elites not involved in the toilet market. For example, are Ng Sang and Li Tak Cheong, who were shareholders of Chinese Insurance Co. In the mid-1870s, Li and two other elites, his uncle Li Sing and toilet landowner Cheng Sing Yeung, bought the company in 1882. Next was Pow Ping Kwan, who joined the toilet market at the end of the decade noted in Chap. 4, who became a major shareholder in subsequent years.[90] In the late 1870s, Pow Ping Kwan also entered into a land business partnership with Ng Sang and Leong On; comprador to Gibbs, Livingston & Company and founding member of PLK and TWH, as shown in Chap. 2.[91] Cheng Sing Yeung also started a similar partnership with another toilet landowner, Tso Wing Yung, and other business elites, such as Li Sing and Li Tak Cheong.[92]

There is much evidence that toilet landowners had social relationships among themselves and with other elites, which intensified as more of these landowners became social leaders through directorships of PLK and TWH, an indication of elite status. Seven toilet landowners were also directors or chairmen of PLK and TWH at some time: Choy Kwai Ng (Choy Chan's son), Hu Tso, Ip Ching Chuen, Kwok Acheong, Ku Fai Shan, Lo Kun Ting and Pow Ping Kwan. For example, toilet landowners Hu Tso and Ng Sang shared a common friend—Ip Chuk Kai—comprador to Reiss & Company, and director of both PLK (1883/4, 1885/6, 1894/5) and TWH (1873/4, 1881/2, 1888/9).[93] Ng Sang appointed Ip as executor in 1883, and in return, Ip appointed Hu in 1901.[94] Meanwhile, Ip himself was also a friend of another two toilet landowners, Ng Ping Sam and Pow Ping Kwan, and all three were partners of Sun On Bank in the 1880s.[95] The company was founded by Li Hong Zhang, the Minister of Beiyang, in 1872, as part of the Self-Strengthening movement to capture international trade in the late Ch'ing dynasty.[96] In addition, two toilet landowners, Ku Fai Shan and Lo Kun Ting, and prominent Chinese elites, such as Ho Kai and the tycoon Ho Tung's younger brother, Ho Fook (Jardine Matheson comprador), formed the Chinese Commercial Union in the late nineteenth century, later changing its name to the Chinese Chamber of Commerce.[97]

From the growing wealth and rising social status of Chinese business elites, a new political order was formed. To foster better government-business relations, some Chinese elites were appointed honorable posts, which highly increased the social interaction of these elites with other elites through regular meetings. Toilet landowner appointments are summarized in Table 5.1. Both Ng Sang and Pow Ping Kwan were appointed to the Committee on Emigration of Women to US in the mid-1870s, which also included Leong On. Another example is Ku Fai Shan, who was an appointee of the Typhoon Relief Fund Committee in the early twentieth century, prominent among its members were Chau Siu Ki, P. Chater, Ho Kai, and H.N. Mody, a distinguished Parsi businessman and land developer.[98] Additionally, was Ho Kam Tong, who was Jardine Matheson & Co.'s comprador and the tycoon Ho Tung's younger brother.[99] From the above examples, it can be seen that toilet operators' relationships with each other and other elites were so networked together through direct and indirect social ties (whereby people are connected by a third party) and through multiple types of interaction (personal, social, business, and political) as stated above that they became a united entity.

Such interweaving of networks increased their influence upon each other and provided the setting for the exchange of obligations, even though some of them were only linked indirectly.[100] Zuo et al. alerts us to the strength of indirect ties connected via multiple interactions on information flows.[101] They find that relationships are stronger when connected through more than one or two types of interaction. The intensity of interaction increases with a higher number of pathways between individuals. Multiple pathways made people more socially close, as they could be 'a friend of many of one's friend', allowing them to influence others indirectly.[102] Their work provides insight into the strengthening effect of multiple types of social interaction that stem from being involved in a densely interconnected social network.

Therefore, multiple indirect ties had the potential for the toilet landowners to affect other elites' decisions, which made the latter more willing to tolerate the negative public nuisances generated by privately owned toilets. By illustrating these landowners' capacity to sustain toilet services using their land holdings and interlocking relationships with other elites, this section shows their role in maintaining urban hygiene over the long term. Without such land holdings and connections to powerful elites, the public toilets, which were the sole sanitation infrastructure for many tenement buildings in the Chinese quarter at the time, would not have been able to function. The strategies used by the landowners successfully addressed toilet complaints, securing the long-term operation of these toilet services. Business owners who held critical land resources were better able to offer the services. Their land enabled them to manage the negative externalities (land scarcity, miasma from toilet) and political jostling (urban contestation from other powerful landowners) that resulted from conflicts between Chinese and European landowners, Chinese politicians, and colonial administrators over the use of urban land. This sharing and devolution of power, to a certain extent, reflected the complex interactions amongst the government and Chinese in the land-centered capitalism of Hong Kong. The consequence, however, was the government's ultimate dependence on toilet landowners for this most basic element of urban governance.

5.4 Conclusion

The presence of night soil profit was the central driver for the commercialization of toilet provision into a means of profit accumulation. This had significant impacts on the spatial logic of sanitation infrastructure in regulating urban space. This chapter discusses the combination of political interventions and economic and social strategies, which were employed by a great variety of actors (government, European inspectors, Chinese business elites, and district watchmen), in maintaining toilet cleanliness and securing toilet economies. Nonetheless, this also involved tension between the actors. Furthermore, negotiations between moral and economic imperatives and the balance of spatial regulation and profit accumulation were inherent in public toilets. This is contrary to viewing urban hygiene as a process completely controlled by the colonial government. It is therefore more fruitful to look at the interplay between different actors and strategies. The reordering of urban space was achieved not only through the legal system and the force of bureaucratic apparatuses but also through Chinese land resources and political social networking.

The shared interests of night soil profit and control over lower-class Chinese bodily waste led businesses and governments to work together. Such cooperation blended moral and capitalist logics in public toilet facilities. Furthermore, the two logics were politically and economically blended in the constant negotiation of urban regulation and profit accumulation that evolved through the public toilet era. In doing so, these moral urban spaces came to simultaneously be sites of the means of production, formulating a new moral geography. Therefore, the regulation of urban space was not solely determined by the colonial authority in reference to colonial-power orthodoxies but rather blended with Chinese business and class interests. As a result, in this complex interaction between the market and regulation, the interests of the government and business were both satisfied. While both government and privately owned public toilets served primarily as night soil collection points, they still played a role in maintaining public health through the operation of a new set of discourses concerning hygiene and were the only sanitation infrastructure present in the Chinese quarter.

Notes

1. Polanyi, 1985: 68.
2. Andrews, 1996; Brunton, 2005.
3. Prejudice to Chinese was easily found in the Colonial Surgeon's reports, for example, the Sanitary Reports (Hong Kong), *AR*, 1879. More about Chinese' inability to self-regulate, see Howell, 2004; Levine, 1998.

4. Chadwick 1882; Hong Kong Government 1899; Public Latrines in Hong Kong, *HKT*, 26 March 1891.
5. Mitchell, 1988.
6. Hong Kong Government, 1899. CRN, HKRS149-2-1181, 1885; HKRS149-2-1415, 1889.
7. For the government toilets, see CRN, HKRS149-2-1181, 1885. For the privately owned toilets, see Hong Kong Government, 1899: 6.
8. Chadwick, 1882: 23.
9. Hong Kong Government, 1899: 10.
10. Chadwick, 1882: 18.
11. Hong Kong Government, 1899: 9.
12. Latrine at Hunghom, *HKH*, 27 February 1902.
13. CRN, HKRS149-2-1251, 1885. More regulations to supervise the works of contractors, see by-laws under the Public Health Ordinance, 1887, *GG*, 23 November, 1889, p.919, 30 November 1889, p. 984; By-laws under the Public Health and Buildings Ordinance, 1903–1909, *GG*, 22 September 1912, p. 565–7.
14. CRN, HKRS149-2-1883, 1898–1901, 149-2-317, 1912; By-laws under the Public Health and Buildings Ordinance, 1903–1909, *GG*, 22 September 1912, p. 565–7.
15. Corbin, 1986; Freud, 1961; Huang, 2016.
16. Chadwick, 1842.
17. Andrews, 1990; Wohl, 1983.
18. Elias, 1939; Freud, 1961.
19. Benedict, 1996; Gilman, 1985; Rogaski 2004.
20. Huang (2016).
21. Ordinance for the Maintenance of Order and Cleanliness, *GG*, 22 June 1867, No.96, p. 231–2; Instructions to the Senior Inspector of Nuisances, Instructions to Inspectors of Nuisances, Instructions to Head Watchmen and Watchmen, *GG*, 23 June 1883, No.223, p. 538–44, 549–51.
22. Levine, 1998.
23. Foucault, 1990.
24. Dean, 1999.
25. Ordinance for the Maintenance of Order and Cleanliness, *GG*, 22 June 1867, No. 96, p. 231–2.
26. Chadwick, 1882: 41.
27. Sanitary Board, *GG*, 21 April 1883, No. 144, p. 363–4.
28. Instructions to Police Officers, GG, 23 June 1883, No. 223, p.5 44.
29. Eitel, 1895: 364, 447–8.
30. Chadwick, 1882: 42.
31. Arnold, 1993; Yeoh, 1996.
32. Sanitary Board, *GG*, 21 April 1883, No. 144, p. 363–4.
33. Chadwick, 1882: 2, 42.
34. Chu, 2013a.
35. Huang, 2016; Kidami, 2007; Rogaski 2004.

36. Chadwick, 1882: 42.
37. Instructions to Inspectors of Nuisances, *GG*, 23 June 1883, No. 223, p. 543; Instructions to Head Watchmen and Watchmen, *GG*, 23 June 1883, No. 223, p. 544.
38. Instructions to the Senior Inspector of Nuisances, *GG*, 23 June 1883, No. 223, p. 538–44.
39. Number and Cost of District Watchmen, *GG*, 27 October 1883, No.345, p. 832.
40. Hamilton, 1998: 208–9.
41. Hamilton, 1998.
42. Hamilton, 1998: 208.
43. Hamilton, 1998.
44. Chadwick, 1882: 5.
45. Hong Kong Government, 1899.
46. Instructions to Inspectors of Nuisances, GG, 23 June 1883, p. 541.
47. Alleged Bribery of Public Servant, SCMP, 23 August 1906.
48. Interpreter to the Inspector of Nuisances, *GG*, 18 February 1882, No. 65, p.181.
49. Inspector of Nuisance, *GG*, 30 November 1878, No.234, p. 582,
50. Inspector of Nuisance, *GG*, 23 June 1883, No. 223, p. 542.
51. Latrines, *GG*, 21 February 1891, No.63, p.124; Report of the Director of Public Works, *AR*, 1913, P53.
52. Report of the Director of Public Works for the year 1918, *AR*, 1918, Q.53.
53. *HKH*, 18 June 1908.
54. Latrine at Wanchai Gap Road, HKRS 203-1-25, 1903.
55. Hong Kong Government, 1899: 4.
56. Chadwick, 1882: 54.
57. Hong Kong Government, 1899: 8–10; Report of the Director of Public Works for the year 1918, *AR*, 1918, Q.53.
58. The contractors were bound by the rules and regulations issued by the Governor in Council under the *1867 Ordinance for the Maintenance of Order and Cleanliness* and the *1883 Order and Cleanliness Amendment Ordinance*, see CRN, HKRS149-2-1247, 1885. The operators were bound by the by-laws specific to toilets made under the *1887 Public Health Ordinance*, see Latrines, *GG*, 21 February 1891, No. 63, p.124.
59. Public Latrines in Hong Kong, *HKT*, 26 March 1891; MSB, *GG*, 22 August, 24 October and 14 November 1891.
60. CRN, HKRS149-2-1181, 1885, HKRS149-2-1883, 1898–1921.
61. Special sanitary service, 22 June 1895, No. 115, p. 758.
62. Plague Epidemic, *GG*, 13 April 1895, p.373. See also the *Report by the Medical Officer of Health*, 1895, p. 353–4.
63. Plague Epidemic, *GG*, 13 April 1895, p. 374.
64. Epidemic of Bubonic Fever, *GG*, 15 December 1900. For the population, see population, *BB*, 1894, M2.

65. Farnham Common, 1996: 130. See also governor's dispatch to the Secretary of State with reference to the plague, *SP*, 20 June 1894, p. 283–92.
66. Special sanitary service, 22 June 1895, No. 115, p. 758.
67. Gough Street Latrine, HKRS202-1-10-6, 1904.
68. CRN, HK149-2-1395, 1889.
69. Lee Ching v. Pang Tai Yuen and Kwong Kam Tong, *CM*, 7 April 1893.
70. Ng Tat Chi v. Chan Pui, *HKWP*, 2 January 1896.
71. Ng Tat Chi v. Chan Pui, *HKWP*, 2 January 1896.
72. Gough Street Latrine, HKRS202-1-10-6, 1904.
73. Criminal Statistics, *SP*, 1880–1910.
74. Hong Kong Government, 1899: 8–10.
75. HKRS38-2, *RB*, 1865–1875.
76. Eitel, 1895.
77. Bankruptcy, *GG*, 15 April and 14 October 1882, 7 July and 4 August 1883, 25 October 1884.
78. Axelrod, 1984.
79. Chan, 1991.
80. Chan, 1991: 115.
81. HKRS38-2, *RB*, 1877–95.
82. Fichtner, 1976: 249.
83. Hu Choo, HKRS144-4-2086, 1908.
84. Tang, 1996. According to Lo (1971), the Tangs also intermarried with Ho Tung's family, unfortunately no evidence was found.
85. CS/I005/00044007.GIF, CS/I005/00044009.GIF, Carl Smith Collection; PLK Archive.
86. Probate, *BB*, 2 February 1888; Tsang Sam, HKRS144-4-689; Lo, 1971.
87. CS/I007/00061845.GIF, CS/I001/00005933.GIF, Carl Smith Collection.
88. Ho Tsoi, *GG*, 28 Oct 1899; CS/I002/00015460.GIF, Carl Smith Collection.
89. Liao, 1973.
90. About Ng and Li, CS/I017/00163159.GIF, CS/I017/00163160.GIF, Carl Smith Collection. For the purchase, CS/I017/00163157.GIF, Carl Smith Collection. About Pow, Tung Wah Hospital, *GG*, 14 July 1883, p. 614.
91. For the land partnership, see M.L.No.140, HKRS 265-11D-2466-1, 1877.
92. CS/I001/00008055.GIF, Carl Smith Collection.
93. CS/I002/00017269.GIF, Carl Smith Collection; PLK Archive, TWH Archive.
94. Ip Chuk Kai, HKRS144-4-2183, 1901; Ng Sang, HKRS144-4-501, 1883.
95. CS/I002/00017271.GIF, CS/I002/00017272.GIF, CS/I004/00036579.GIF, CS/I004/00038075.GIF, Carl Smith Collection.
96. For the company. see Reinhardt, 2007. For Yung's profile, see CS/I006/00054285.GIF, Carl Smith Collection; TWH Archive.
97. About Ho Fook, see CS/I004/00037989.GIF, Carl Smith Collection. About the Chamber, see Chan, 1956; Zhang, 2012.
98. Report of the Typhoon Relief Fund Committee, *GG*, 17 May 1907, p. 246. About the elites, see Carroll, 2007; Mellor, 1992.
99. CS/I002/00014849.GIF, Carl Smith Collection.

100. Burt, 1987; Zuo et al., 2015.
101. Zuo et al., 2015.
102. Zuo et al., 2015: 188.

Chapter 6
Concluding Remarks: A Moral-Capitalist Mode of Urban Governance of Public Toilets

6.1 Overview

The purely political analysis of public toilets in colonies has generally emphasized the moral claim to civilize the local population and thereby promote the hygienic need to regulate their bodies. The analysis in this book extends the political framework by analyzing the creation and management of toilets as both a political and economic space in colonial Hong Kong. Throughout the second half of the nineteenth century, the broad and deep influence of the world economy became an everyday reality as public toilets were operated as night soil collection points. This brought complex interactions between key players in the colony (governor, colonial administrators, European landowners, and Chinese landowners and politicians) embedded within racial (colonial governance of lower-class Chinese) and class (characterized by economic interests) politics in the regulation and profit accumulation of urban space. The political and economic interactions that occurred over public toilets challenged the perceived spatial order of colonial authority. That the toilets functioned as both a moral space and as a means of production meant that they not only blended moral and economic logics but also racial and class politics in a capitalist system, producing a new moral geography. This discussion identified two dominant forces: the primary fear of environmental and moral threat, that disease originating from lower-class Chinese bodily waste threatened the integrity of the colony, and the profitability of "toilet economies". These forces together supported an urban governance arrangement between the government and Chinese business elites, which came to shape the development of sanitation infrastructure. Employed was a moral-capitalist mode of urban governance, based on a particular set of regulations and interests, to achieve the regulation of urban space in a capitalist-colonial context, bound up with the colonial economy and world system.

Y. Chong, *Toilet as Business for the Hygiene of the Chinese Community in Colonial Hong Kong*, https://doi.org/10.1007/978-981-19-1396-9_6

6.2 Dynamics of Resource Exchange Between Government and Business

With the power of land, manpower, wealth and social-political capital, the Chinese elites' role in Hong Kong was not that of passive recipients. The notion of colonial modernization rested on a hegemony of a civilizing project that catered to the needs of colonies by promising to build a civilized and moral rationality, putting the colonizer and colonized into a vertical framework of guardian and child.[1] However, the business elites who accumulated great land and wealth were able to develop their abilities to become potential, and then real, partners in providing public services and maintaining security, usurping racial guardian-child hegemony, as Chap. 2 "Political-Economic Conditions for Chinese Business Elites Taking a Role in Governance" describes. The collaboration was founded on resource exchange between the government and business in that they needed the resources of each other to achieve their respective goals. For the government, the elites were gradually coopted into colonial governance, offering much-needed services to general Chinese as well as maintaining the law and order of the colony, which helped sustain colonial rule. For business, their political and economic power and social position were enhanced through delivering public services and participating in the daily operation of the colony.

Weiss describes this type of collaboration as "governed interdependence", where both the government and the private sector have strong resource capacity but in different aspects that are conducive to exchange, making public–private collaboration possible.[2] She argues that the two parties could negotiate the relationship and maintain cooperation as long as they are interdependent on each other's resources. However, it is hard to say which party captures the other or which submits to the other. As we saw, this was the case in early Hong Kong, where the control of resources by business enabled resource exchange, which facilitated urban governance between the colonial government and Chinese business in reordering urban space through the provision of public toilets. Both government and business were equipped with particular resources that the other lacked but needed. The business provided and sustained toilet services by huge land resources and a team of night soil coolies that helped maintain urban hygiene. Meanwhile, the government offered pro-Chinese business measures (e.g., no requirement of night soil disinfection) based on laws and conferred political appointments upon them. That resource interdependence sustained government-business urban governance, implying that their relations were not anchored at two extremes.[3] Their interactions were therefore drastically altered from being binary and hierarchical along racial lines to a more interactive and collaborative relationship. The result was that the vertical political structure of colonial rule was challenged, allowing Chinese business to transcend the colonizer-colonized and public–private dichotomies of colonial governance.

This strengthened their respective bargaining power with each other. A negotiated relationship was maintained as long as government and business were interdependent for resources. The relationship can be better understood as collaborative while also being competitive, for example was business' continual negotiation and renegotiation of the goals and policies of public health proposals in 1856, 1878, 1887 and 1891, as discussed in Chap. 3, "Governing Urban Space: Racial and Class Politics". Examining the capitalist dimension of public health proposals and toilet provision in colonial Hong Kong illuminates the operation of colonial economies and the formation of discourses of sanitation infrastructure. Urban hygiene should not be treated as sets of relations outside of the market economy but rather emerges out of the tensions and contradictions between urban regulation and profit accumulation of urban space. As shown in this chapter, the contestation by Chinese business (allied with Chinese politicians, European landowners and administration officials) over the use of space was integrated with the new economic opportunities (high land prices) that arose out of dramatic changes to the economic system of the region. This is apparent in the rapid rise in political and economic power of the business elites, who felt confident enough to challenge the orthodox moral discourse of urban hygiene and provide public toilets themselves.

Indeed, the collaboration between the government and business elites often involved contestation over the usage of urban land. Business tended to use its links with Chinese politicians such as Ho Kai to contest the meanings of sanitation infrastructure while arguing that the infrastructure as a means of production was governed by the logic of profit making within a capitalist system. On the other hand, in consideration of its own political agenda in 1890, the government using its political authority urgently passed the by-laws about public toilets to empower it by reinstating control over the running of privately owned public toilets. This move indicated that the government had not surrendered to the business sector and could maintain negotiation through its monopoly of legal power of licensing. These movements from the government and business show the tensions and contradictions of a form of urban regulation that was engaged with profit accumulation of urban space while embedded in a colonial capitalist system. This created the conditions for the capitalist turn of public toilets.

6.3 Tying Colonial Sanitation to the Global Consumer Silk Market

Well aware of the rising demand for night soil as part of the vibrant silk industry in Shunde, the economic sensitivity of Hong Kong Chinese business elites (night soil contractors, toilet operators, and toilet landowners) to the potential night soil profits drove a dramatic change in the colony's public toilet landscape from the late 1860s, as shown in Chap. 4, "Toilet Economies: Night Soil Profit, Entrance Fee and Rent". On a global scale, the colonial economic system was highly centered on the West. Through creating demand for commodities, global economic forces had a strong impact on the balance of urban governance between the government and business owners. Under this circumstance, toilet as a night soil collection point was exposed to global colonial economic restructuring of areas of silk consumption, mechanization of silk manufacturing and inequalities of areas for primarily resource extraction (raw silk). Night soil markets connected the Hong Kong public toilets to China's silk industry, which in turn was significantly influenced by global consumer silk demand and the world system of peripheral areas that supplied raw silk for the core economies. This meant that the demand for night soil was tied to that of silk.

The connections between colonial sanitation, global capitalist silk markets and night soil run deep. While public toilets and the surrounding countryside did complement each other's purposes, one providing fertilizer and the other a sustainable income, the global economic linkages between the world silk market, China's silk industry and the Hong Kong night soil business opened original economic opportunities. The presence of such opportunities created strong economic incentives for both the government and business to work hand-in-hand to collect night soil for profit and continue operating marketized toilet services. The result was a citywide network of commercial public toilets that served as night soil collection points for a cross-border market of night soil collection and trade within the world silk industry. Being operated in a market-centered manner, the prevalence and breadth of toilet services became to be determined by market forces. The economic sustainability and rationale of toilet services were highly dependent on the dynamics of these new global markets and economic centers. Within the world system, market-driven toilet provision was linked to China's silk industry and world silk demand, putting toilet provision at the mercy of world market forces. This meant that public toilets became economically sustainable when night soil demand grew, which occurred regionally as the silk industry in nearby Shunde rapidly developed through the nineteenth century. Furthermore, business withdrew from the toilet market during the decline of the world silk market of the Great Depression.

Furthermore, capitalist markets introduced into colonial management an aspect of maximization of interests that led to the intensive use of urban space as commercial public toilets, complicating the spatial regulation by the government that was imposed on the general Chinese population and creating a new mode of economic behavior into urban governance (noted in Chap. 2). However, in parallel, colonial rule was devised around the idea of minimal government; as such, it avoided intervention in Chinese daily life to prevent conflict, and this nonintervention was a supportive force for capitalist expansion. It is true that worries about disease transmission were a major factor shaping the government to work with Chinese business elites over the regulation of urban space. Such a style of governing led to market-driven service provision in which the availability of toilets was left to market forces operating on local, regional and global scales in the world system. Thus, in a capitalist context such as Hong Kong, it is not surprising that public toilet development became implemented in line with profit maximization. Before 1899, the toilet business was mainly dominated by Chinese business elites, especially landed class elites; thus, we can infer that they played a decisive role in urban hygiene. The formative importance of land ownership and land resources suggests that these were critical factors in the urban governance of public toilets. This allowed the colonial government to remain a minimal government; indeed, as Lau notes, a condition for minimal government to succeed was that the local "society is resourceful enough to deal with its salient problems".[4] Therefore, by providing the necessary resources (land, night coolies) to establish and sustain public toilet services, Chinese business facilitated the government to collaborate in toilet provision.

It is argued that in a context full of racial and class contention, a consent-based model of collaboration is applicable to colonial Hong Kong. As shown in Chap. 5, "A Blending of Moral and Capitalist Logics in Public Toilets", Chinese elites and the government were not partnering in all aspects, and tended to opt-in or opt-out without much hesitation, their relationship was indicative of one of consent, rather than formal collaboration. It is critical to realize that collaboration by consent is much less committed than formal collaboration.[5] It must be noted that, as Kavanagh and Morris describe, consent is "*a set of parameters which bounded the set of policy options regarded by senior politicians and civil servants as administratively practicable, economically affordable and politically acceptable* (italics original)".[6] Collaboration by consent is made possible through using a mutual scope of understanding, thereby imposing a kind of obligation on the parties involved that requires them to respond in an expected way. It can be said that consent is only viable when collaborators clearly understand that they are mutually interdependent. As government-business cooperation in public toilets did not rely on formal collaborative structures but rather on consent—informal interactions with tacit mutual understanding—both parties understood they were mutually interdependent. With this understanding, they were bound by certain parameters. First, as long as business sustained toilet services, then their interests (night soil profit and rental) would be protected, in that the government would maintain the pail system through introducing pro-business measures (no disinfection requirement to night soil deposited in toilets), supervising the daily night soil removal and toilet operation, and through enacting the *Latrine Ordinance* in 1891 that restricted competitors from entering the toilet market. Furthermore, the provision of privately owned toilets minimized the necessity of government toilets. In tandem, Chinese business owners understood their responsibility to remove night soil daily, contain toilet complaints and sustain toilet services.

As consent is less visible and more loosely structured than formal collaboration, it does not always lead to consensus and harmony. Conflicts of interest are possible even in the consent mode of collaboration. Kavanagh and Morris remind us that under a consent model, disagreements are merely contained and not solved, and therefore, the terms of collaboration could change when disagreements are no longer successfully suppressed.[7] It is true that the disagreements between the Hong Kong colonial government and Chinese business elites over the deodorization of night soil were merely contained, and this containment was the result of a rational calculation of interests—the manurial value of night soil (a key factor of the continuing toilet service), as seen in Chap. 5. Night soil demand depended on manurial value, and the business sector strategically made use of this hard reality to press the government to exercise its authority by relaxing disinfection requirements in privately owned public toilets. Functional dependence on these toilets drove the government to compromise the deodorization requirement unless there was a public health crisis.

Furthermore, colonial collaboration was always a strategic equilibrium interwoven with complex racial and class tension, adding unstable elements to it, making it inherently fragile and unstable, which was reflected in their opted-in and opted-out, as shown in Chaps. 3, 4 and 5.[8] For example, the inherent instability can be seen in the cases discussed in this chapter, whereby fear of disease contamination of general Chinese on Europeans, night soil and land interests moved the government and business together, while the decline of night soil demand split their interests, resulting in business withdrawal from the toilet market. The terms of collaboration changed as the terms of their interests shifted, while the status of the collaboration needed to be frequently reconfirmed. Clearly, the relationship between the colonial government and Chinese business owners over toilet provision was built on a very strong common self-interest in urban space. Nonetheless, they were by no means committed to each other and had no guaranteed obligation to smooth over conflicts of interest. Their relationship was dynamic; they were not serving each other's interests but only collaborated at certain points according to their own needs, as noted in various chapters. As we have seen in the interplay between the business elites' constraint of government-owned toilets, facilitation of privately owned toilets due to profit. Meanwhile, the government relaxed the night soil disinfection requirement due to the manurial value of night soil. It can be said that the public toilets mediated the interests and relations between the government and business owners, and they brought about a new strategic collaboration of commodifying the toilets as a means of production, actualizing and constituting each other's moral and economic interests, creating a capitalist-political turn of sanitation.

Business owners who held critical land resources were better able to offer toilet services. Their land enabled them to manage the negative externalities (land scarcity, miasma from toilet) and political jostling (urban contestation from other powerful landowners) that resulted from conflicts between Chinese and European landowners, Chinese politicians, and colonial administrators over the use of urban land. This sharing and devolution of power, to a certain extent, reflected the complex interactions amongst the government and Chinese in the land-centered capitalism of Hong Kong, as Chap. 5 shows.

6.4 A New Moral Geography: Sanitary Infrastructure and Business Venture

The prevailing ethnic-colonial spatial relations were particularly contested when capitalism, then centered on estate property development, provided a source of power that granted Chinese business a privileged political and civil position. With large land holdings, business owners could strategically support public toilet services through the use of their "spheres of influence", as Chap. 5 shows. In doing so, Chinese landowners freed the government of the difficulty of finding appropriate toilet sites and managing complaints in the already densely populated colony. As huge land resources were necessary for the spheres of influence to be possible, the government was driven to adopt more lenient views toward toilet sanitary standards, as long as the toilet site could contain public complaints and continue to provide toilet services. When used as a tool to provide public toilets, the control of land became political in that it allowed business to solve economic (fiscal constraints, land scarcity) and political (toilet site negotiations from other powerful landowners, and intervention in Chinese's daily life) problems for the government, which at the time had limited land resources, manpower and money to adequately provide and sustain toilet services in the medium to long term. To secure their economic interests, business owners were dependent on government efforts to provide pro-business measures (e.g., tax incentives) that nurtured the conditions essential for private interest to enter the toilet market and ensure a vertically integrated inspector and legal system, which helped ensure toilet services were sustainable in terms of hygiene. This echoes what Polanyi argues in this chapter that regulation and the market interact with each other and develop together.

Managed in collaboration by the government and business, the public toilets became a negotiated space between profit and morality. For the government, the toilets exercised a moral function of regulating public defecation and helping enforce colonial spatial order, a designated use-pattern of urban space that was moral space. For business, toilets were commercial ventures, and thus, their spatial organization was guided by maximizing the collection of night soil. Therefore, they were most common in the Chinese quarter, where residential buildings lacked domestic toilets. This was also important to relieve the business pressure to provide domestic toilets to their tenants through public toilet provision. In this balance of interests, we see the ability of business to work with the government to reshape land use in response to profit-seeking and spatial regulation so that the spatial technology of profitable night soil collection points was developed. The result was that the spatial ordering of toilet space was arranged according to the logic of profit, differing from the colonial government's ideal moral spatial order. Profit significantly impacted the regulation of urban space, undermining the old moral geography of colonizer British and colonized Chinese. The public toilets were not derived simply from a discursive ethnic-moral order: dirty Chinese and clean British, but rather were driven by both moralist and capitalist concerns.

It can be said that commercial public toilets (both government-owned and privately owned) were a byproduct of a combination of conditions: first, the fear of disease and contamination of European morality due to frequent disease outbreaks, second, a prosperous land-centered and capitalist economy, and third, the rapid development of the silk industry in the Pearl River Delta, under the influence of the world silk market. This demonstrates the complex historical interplay of political-economic conditions, which were marked by the dynamics of regulation and profit accumulation of urban space, which guided the government and dominant nongovernment players, especially landowners, to construct a citywide network of public toilets. The collective provision of the toilets reflects how "toilet economics" generated significant political consequences, allowing business to play a greater role in urban governance. Chinese business owners not only exploited the new opportunities that the government and land-centered capitalism had presented but also reshaped the public health logic of the regulation of space and the nature of sanitation infrastructure so that it had to accommodate private economic interests.

To summarize, this analysis contributes to a new understanding of colonial health policies, urban governance and sanitary infrastructure and gives new impetus to exploring how the commercial potential of public toilets might create multiple economic logics that turn these facilities into overlapping moral-economic spaces. As toilets overlap the goals of profit accumulation and the regulation of space, satisfying both government and business interests, those interests were not necessarily opposed. This helps explain how urban governance works in a capitalist climate, involving complex interactions between capitalism, morality and urban space. Such an outcome not only implied that public toilet services did not necessarily need to be provided solely by the government but also indicated that morality alone was not enough to achieve the regulation of urban space, so the government had to take into account business interests. Overall, it can be seen that the capitalist-moral mode of urban governance of public toilets was far more effective in addressing toilet service sustainability than a purely moral mode. While the toilets primarily operated as night soil collection points, through the operation of a new set of hygiene and profit (toilets as a means of production) discourses, they played a major role in public health by containing human waste and moralizing lower-class Chinese bodies. This made the public toil the product of both regulation and profit accumulation derived from urban space, bringing a new moral geography to Hong Kong.

Notes

1. Cain, 2012; Crowder, 1970; Curtin, 1964; Woolf, 1928.
2. Weiss, 1998.
3. Block and Evans, 1994; Ngo, 1999, Weiss, 1988.
4. Lau, 1982: 19.
5. Pierre and Peters, 2000.
6. Kavanagh and Morris, 1989: 13.
7. Kavanagh and Morris, 1989.
8. Chan, 1991; Tsai, 1993.

References

1. Anderson W (1995) Excremental Colonialism: public health and the poetics of pollution. Crit Inq 21(3):640–669
2. Andrews MW (1990) Sanitary conveniences and the retreat of the frontier: vancouver, 1886–1926. BC Stud 87:3–22
3. Arnold D (1993) Colonizing the body: state medicine and epidemic disease in nineteenth-century India. University of California Press, Berkeley
4. Arnold D (1994) Public health and public power: medicine and hegemony in colonial India. In: Engels D, Marks S (eds) Contesting colonial hegemony: state and society in Africa and India. The German Historical Institute, London, London & New York, pp 131–151
5. Axelrod R (1984) The evolution of cooperation. Basic Books, New York
6. Barcan R (2010) Dirty spaces: separation, concealment, and shame in the public toilet. In: Molotch H, Norén L (eds) Public restrooms and the politics of sharing. NYU Press, New York, pp 25–41
7. Bashford A (1998) Purity and pollution: gender, embodiment and victorian medicine. Macmillan Press, Houndmills, Basingstoke, Hampshire and London, St. Martin's Press, New York
8. Baverman I (2010) Potty training: nonhuman inspection in public washrooms. In: Molotch H, Norén L (eds) Public restrooms and the politics of sharing. NYU Press, New York, pp 65–86
9. Benedict C (1996) Bubonic plague in nineteenth-century China. Stanford University Press, California
10. Bhabha HK (1994) The location of culture. Routledge, London and New York
11. Block F, Evans P (1994) The state and the economy. In: Smelser NJ, Swedberg R (eds) The handbook of economic sociology. Princeton University Press, Princeton, pp 505–526
12. Bristow R (1984) Land-use planning in Hong Kong: history, policies and procedures. Oxford University Press, Hong Kong
13. Brunton D (2005) Evil necessaries and abominable erections: public conveniences and private interests in the Scottish City, 1830–1870. Soc Hist Med 18(2):187–202
14. Burt RS (1987) Social contagion and innovation: cohesion versus structural equivalence. Am J Sociol 92(6):1287–1335
15. Cain PJ (2012) Character, 'Ordered Liberty', and the mission to civilize: british moral justification of empire, 1870–1914. J Imp Commonw Hist 557–578
16. Cain PJ, Hopkins AG (1993) British imperialism: innovation and expansion, 1688–1914. Longman, London and New York
17. Carnoy M (1984) The state and political theory. Princeton University Press, New Jersey
18. Carroll JM (2007) Edge of empires: chinese elites and British colonials in Hong Kong. Hong Kong University Press, Hong Kong

Y. Chong, *Toilet as Business for the Hygiene of the Chinese Community in Colonial Hong Kong*, https://doi.org/10.1007/978-981-19-1396-9

19. Chadwick E (1842) Report on the sanitary condition of the labouring population of great britain. Routledge/Thaoemmes Press, London
20. Chadwick E (1997) Public health. Routledge/Thoemmes Press, London, Sanitation and its Reform
21. Chadwick O (1882) Mr. Chadwick's report on the sanitary condition of Hong Kong. Hong Kong Government Printers, Hong Kong
22. Chan WK (1991) The making of Hong Kong society: three studies of class formation in early Hong Kong. Clarendon Press, Oxford
23. Chapman SD (1971) The history of working-class housing. David and Charles, Newton Abbot
24. Chattopadhyay S (2005) Representing calcutta: modernity, nationalism, and the colonial uncanny. Routledge, London and New York
25. Chen XP (1941) The revolutionary history of the revive china society. Chinese Culture Service Agency, China
26. Choa GH (1981) The life and times of Sir Kai Ho Kai. Chinese University Press, Hong Kong
27. Choi YC (1999) The dynamics of public service contracting: the British experience. Policy Press, Bristol
28. Chu C (2013) Combating nuisance: sanitation, regulation, and the politics of property in colonial Hong Kong. In: Peckham R, Pomfret DM (eds) Imperial contagions: medicine, hygiene, and cultures of planning in Asia. Hong Kong University Press, Hong Kong, pp 17–36
29. Chu C (2013) Shanzheng and gongde: moral regulation and narratives of 'Good Government' in Colonial Hong Kong. J Hist Geogr 42:180–192
30. Coates A (1980) Whampoa: ships on the shore. South China Morning Post, Hong Kong
31. Corbin A (1986) The foul and the fragrant: odor and the french social imagination. Harvard University Press, Cambridge
32. Cowell C (2013) The Hong Kong fever of 1843: collective trauma and the reconfiguration of colonial space. Mod Asian Stud 47:329–354
33. Crowder M (1970) West Africa under colonial rule. Hutchinson of London, London
34. Curtin PD (1964) The image of Africa: British ideas and action, 1780–1850. The University of Wisconsin Press, USA
35. Dean M (1999) Governmentality: power and rule in modern society. Sage Publication, London
36. Douglas M (1970) Purity and danger: an analysis of concepts of pollution and taboo. Penguin, Harmondworth
37. Driver F (1988) Moral geographies: social science and the Urban environment in mid-nineteenth century England. Trans Inst Br Geogr 13(3):275–287
38. Eitel EJ (1895) Europe in China: the history of Hong Kong from the beginning to the year 1882. Oxford University Press, Hong Kong
39. Elias N (1939) The civilizing process: the history of manners. Basil Blackwell, Oxford
40. Endacott GB (1964) A history of Hong Kong. Oxford University Press, Hong Kong
41. Eng YY (1986) Imperialism and the Chinese economy: the canton and Shanghai silk industry, 1861–1932. University Microfilms International, Michigan
42. Esherick JW, Rankin MB (1990) Chinese local elites and patterns of dominance. University of California Press, Berkeley
43. Evans DE (1970) Chinatown in Hong kong: the beginnings of Taipingshan. J R Asiatic Soc Hong Kong Branch 12:69–78
44. Evans RJ (1987) Death in hamburg: society and politics in the cholera years, 1830–1910. Clarendon Press, Oxford
45. Ferguson DT (2014) Nightsoil and the 'Great Divergence': human waste, the Urban economy, and economic productivity, 1500–1900. J Glob Hist 9(3):379–402
46. Fichtner PS (1976) Dynasty marriage in sixteenth-century habsburg diplomacy and statecraft: an interdisciplinary approach. Am Hist Rev 81(2):243–265
47. Foucault M (1980) Power/knowledge: selected interviews and other writings, 1972–1977. Vintage Books, New York

48. Foucault M (1990) The history of sexuality. In: Hurley R (trans) An introduction. Vintage Book, New York
49. Freud S (1961) Civilization and its discontents. Norton, New York & London
50. Gandy M (2006) The bacteriological city and its discontents. Hist Geogr 34:14–25
51. Gilman SL (1985) Difference and pathology: stereotypes of sexuality, race, and madness. Cornell University Press, Ithaca
52. Glasco B (2010) Constructing Mexico City: colonial conflicts over cultures, space, and authority. Palgrave Macmillan, New York
53. Goodstadt LF (2005) Uneasy partners: the conflict between public interest and private profit in Hong Kong. Hong Kong University Press, Hong Kong
54. Guangdong Province Chorography (2004) Si Chou Zhi, Vol. 1. Guangdong People's Publishing House, GuangZhou
55. Guangzhou City Chorography Office (1995) Socio-economic situations of contemporary Guangzhou Port. Jinan University Press, Guangzhou
56. Hamilton S (1998) The district watch force. J Hong Kong Branch R Asiatic Soc 38:199–228
57. Hamlin C (1998) Public health and social justice in the age of Chadwick: britain, 1900–1854. Cambridge University Press, Cambridge
58. Harvey D (1982) The limits to capital. Basil Blackwell, Oxford
59. Holdsworth M, Munn C (2012) Dictionary of Hong Kong biography. Hong Kong University Press, Hong Kong
60. Hong Kong Government (1887) Report from the land commission of 1886–1887. Government Printers, Hong Kong
61. Hong Kong Government (1899) Report on the urine and urinal accommodation of the city. Government Printers, Hong Kong
62. Howell P (2004) Race, space and the regulation of prostitution in colonial Hong Kong. Urban Hist 31(2):229–248
63. Huang XL (2016) Deodorizing China: odour, ordure, and colonial (dis)order in Shanghai, 1840s–1940s. Mod Asian Stud 50(3):1092–1222
64. Hui PK (1997) The development of Hong Kong Chinese business in the mid-19th to the early 20th century: a transnational perspective. China Inform 7(1/2)
65. Jackson L (2014) Dirty old London: the Victorian fight against filth. Yale University Press, New Haven
66. Kavanagh D, Morris P (1989) Consensus politics from Attlee to Thatcher. Basil Blackwell, Oxford
67. Kidambi P (2007) The making of an Indian metropolis: colonial Governance and Public Culture in Bombay, 1870–1920. Ashgate, UK
68. King FH (1911) Farmers of forty centuries, or, permanent Agriculture in China, Korea and Japan. Mrs. F. H. King, Madison, Wis
69. Laporte D (2000) History of shit. MIT Press, Cambridge, Mass
70. Lau SK (1982) Society and politics in Hong Kong. The Chinese University Press, Hong Kong
71. Lau WL (2006) Overseas silk trade of contemporary Guangdong. Chung Hwa Books Ltd., Beijing
72. Lau YW (2002) A history of the municipal councils of Hong Kong, 1883–1999: from the sanitary board to the Urban Council. Hong Kong Leisure and Cultural Services Department, Hong Kong
73. Law WS (2009) Collaborative colonial power: the making of the Hong Kong Chinese. Hong Kong University Press, Hong Kong
74. Lefebvre H (1991) In: Nicholson-Smith D (trans) The production of space. Blackwell, Oxford
75. Legg S (2007) Spaces of colonialism: Delhi's Urban governmentalities. Blackwell, Malden
76. Lethbridge HJ (1978) Hong Kong: stability and change: a collection of essay. Oxford University Press, Hong Kong
77. Levine P (1998) Modernity, medicine and colonialism: the contagious diseases ordinances in Hong Kong and the straits settlements. In: Burton A (ed) Gender, sexuality and colonial modernities. Routledge, London and New York, pp 35–48

78. Li M (1981) China's silk trade: traditional industry in the modern world, 1842–1937. Harvard University, Cambridge, Mass, Council on East Asian Studies
79. Li PC (1999) The demand for fertilizer in the Jiangnan region during the Ming-Qing period. Qing Shi Yan Jiu 1(30–38):108
80. Liao MX (1973) Liao mengxing. ChaoYang Publishing Company, Hong Kong
81. Lindblom CE (1977) Politics and markets: the world's political-economic systems. Basic Books, New York
82. Lo HL (1971) Masonry and the development of Hong Kong. Shiu Huo Monthly 1(9):459–463
83. Logan JR, Molotch HL (1987) Urban fortunes: the political economy of place. University of California Press, Berkeley
84. Macpherson K (1987) A wilderness of marshes: the origins of public health in Shanghai, 1843–1893. Oxford University Press, Hong Kong, Oxford and New York
85. Manderson L (1996) Sickness and the state: health and illness in colonial Malaya, 1870–1940. Cambridge University Press, Hong Kong
86. Mcfarlane C (2008) Governing the contaminated city: infrastructure and sanitation in colonial and postcolonial Bombay. Int J Urban Reg Res 32(2):415–425
87. Melosi MV (2000) The Sanitary City: Urban infrastructure in America from colonial times to the present. The John Hopkins University Press, Baltimore and London
88. Melosi MV (2005) Garbage in the cities: refuse, reform, and the environment. University of Pittsburgh Press, USA
89. Migdal JS (1988) Strong societies and weak states: state-society relations and state capabilities in the third world. Princeton University Press, New Jersey
90. Miliband R (1969) The state in capitalist society: the analysis of the western system of power. Quarter Books Limited, London
91. Mills LA (1942) British rule in eastern Asia: a study of contemporary state and economic development in British Malaya and Hong Kong. Oxford University Press, London
92. Mitchell Y (1988) Colonising Egypt. Cambridge University Press, Cambridge
93. Munn C (2009) Anglo-China: Chinese people and British rule in Hong Kong, 1841–1880. Hong Kong University Press, Hong Kong
94. Ngo TW (1999) Colonialism and Hong Kong Revisited. In: Ngo TW (ed) Hong Kong's history: state and society under colonial rule. Routledge, London and New York, pp 1–12
95. Norton-Kyshe JW (1971) The history of the laws and courts of Hong Kong. Vetch and Lee Limited, Hong Kong
96. Parkin F (1971) Class, in class inequality and political order: social stratification in capitalist and communist societies. Praeger, New York
97. Pennell WV (1961) History of the Hong Kong general chamber of commerce, 1861–1961. Cathay Press, Hong Kong
98. Pierre J (2011) The politics of Urban governance. Palgrave Macmillan, Houndmills, Basingstoke, Hampshire, New York
99. Pierre J, Peters BG (2000) Governance. Macmilian Press Ltd., London, Politics and the State
100. Polanyi K (1985) The great transformation. Beacon Press, Boston
101. Pomfret D (2013) "Beyond Risk of Contagion": childhood, hill stations, and the planning of British and French colonial cities. In: Peckham R, Pomfret DM (eds) Imperial contagions: medicine, hygiene, and cultures of planning in Asia. Hong Kong University Press, Hong Kong, pp 81–104
102. Prashad V (2001) The technology of sanitation in colonial Delhi. Mod Asian Stud 35(1):13–155
103. Rear J (1971) One brand of politics. In: Hopkins K (ed) Hong Kong: the industrial colony—A political, social and economic survey. Oxford University Press, Hong Kong, pp 55–139
104. Robinson R (1972) Non-European foundations of european imperialism: sketch for a theory of collaboration. In: Owen ERJ, Sutcliffe RB (eds) Studies in the theory of imperialism. Longman, Bristol, pp 117–142
105. Rogaski R (2004) Hygienic modernity: meanings of health and disease in treaty-port China. University of California Press, Berkeley

106. Scott D (1995) Colonial governmentality. Social Text 43:191–220
107. Shannon TR (1989) An introduction to the world-system perspective. Westview Press, Boulder, Colo
108. Sinn E (2003) Power and charity: a Chinese Merchant Elite in Colonial Hong Kong. Hong Kong University Press, Hong Kong
109. Smith CT (1971) The emergence of a Chinese Elite in Hong Kong. Journal of the Royal Asiatic Society Hong Kong Branch 11:74–115
110. Smith CT (1985) Chinese Christians: Elites, middlemen, and the church in Hong Kong. Oxford University Press, Hong Kong
111. So Y (1986) The South China silk district: local historical transformation and world-system theory. State University of New York Press, Albany
112. Stone CN (1993) Urban regimes and the capacity to govern: a political economy approach. J Urban Aff 15(1):1–28
113. Swanson MW (1977) The sanitation syndrome: bubonic plague and Urban native policy in the Cape colony, 1900–1909. J Afr Hist 18(3):387–410
114. Symons JC (1996) Looking for the stars. Pegasus, Hong Kong
115. Tang KY (1996) My Father Tang Man Chiu. Wen Shi Press Beijing
116. The Commercial Press (1936) Shen's book on agriculture. The Commercial Press, Shanghai
117. Thompson EP (1983) Class consciousness. In: Neale RS (ed) History and class. Basil Blackwell, Oxford, pp 114–142
118. Tobin BF (1999) Picturing imperial power: colonial subjects in eighteenth-century painting. Duke University Press, Durham, N.C
119. Trocki CA (2006) Singapore: wealth, power and the culture of control. Routledge, Oxon
120. Tsai JF (1993) Hong Kong in Chinese history: community and social unrest in the British colony: 1842–1913. Columbia University Press, New York
121. Tung Wah Hospital (1970) One hundred years of the Tung Wah hospitals, 1870–1970. Tung Wah Hospital, Hong Kong
122. Wallerstein I (2004) World-systems analysis: an introduction. Duke University Press, Durham
123. Weiss L (1998) The myth of the powerless state. Polity Press, Cambridge
124. Wohl AS (1983) Endangered lives: public health in victorian britain. Harvard University Press, Cambridge and Massachusetts
125. Wong C (2017) The history of silk industry in the late Qing Dynasty. Shanghai Remin Chubanshe, Shanghai
126. Woolf L (1928) Imperialism and civilization. Harcourt, Brace and Company, New York
127. Wright L (1966) Clean and decent: the fascinating history of the bathroom & the water closet and of sundry habits, fashions & accessories of the toilet, principally in Britain. France & America. Routledge & Kegan Paul, London
128. Xu T (1994) The commodity economy and modernization of Pearl River delta after the Opium War. Qing Shi Yan Jiu 3:70–78
129. Xue Y (2005) "Treasure Nightsoil as If It Were Gold:" economic and ecological links between Urban and Rural areas in late imperial Jiangnan. Late Imperial China 26(1):41–71
130. Yan X (2015) In search of power and credibility essays on Chinese monetary history (1851–1945). Unpublished Ph.D. thesis, The London School of Economics and Political Science
131. Yeoh SA (1996) Contesting space: power relations and the Urban built environment in colonial Singapore. Oxford University Press, Kuala Lumpur
132. Yip KC (2009) Colonialism, disease, and public health: Malaria in the history of Hong Kong. In: Yip KC (ed) Disease, colonialism, and the state: Malaria in modern east Asian history. Hong Kong University Press, Hong Kong, pp 11–30
133. Yu XZ (2010) The treatment of nightsoil and waste in modern China. In: Leung KC, Furth C (eds) Health and hygiene in Chinese East Asia: policies and publics in the long twentieth century. Duke University Press, Durham and London, pp 51–72
134. Yu XZ (2014) Qingdai Jiangnan de Wenyi Yu Shehui Yixiang Yilial Shehuishi de Yanjin. Beijing Normal University Publishing Group, Beijing
135. Zuo X, Blackburn J, Kourtellis N, Skvoretz J, Iamnitchi A (2016) The power of indirect ties. Comput Commun 73:188–199

The manufacturer's authorised representative in the EU is Springer Nature Customer Service Centre GmbH, Europaplatz 3, 69115 Heidelberg, Germany. If you have any concerns regarding our products, please contact ProductSafety@springernature.com

Printed and bound by CPI Group (UK) Ltd, Croydon, CR0 4YY
05/10/2026
02228339-0001